Sacred Space

O servant, where dost thou seek me?
Lo! I am beside thee.
I am neither in the temple nor in the mosque,
    neither am I in rites and ceremonies
    nor in yoga nor in renunciation.
If thou are a true seeker, thou shalt at once see me.
Thou shalt meet me in a moment's time.

The Kabir

For Churchill Livingstone:

Publishing Manager, Health Sciences: Inta Ozols
Head of Project Management: Ewan Halley
Project Development Manager: Valerie Dearing
Designer: Judith Wright/George Ajayi

Sacred Space
Right Relationship and Spirituality in Healthcare

Stephen G Wright RN RCNT DipN DANS MSc RPTT FRCN MBE
Associate Professor, St Martin's College, Lancaster, UK; Chair, The Sacred Space Foundation, Cumbria, UK

Jean Sayre-Adams MA RN
Director, The Sacred Space Foundation, Cumbria, UK

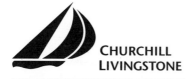

CHURCHILL
LIVINGSTONE

EDINBURGH   LONDON   NEW YORK   PHILADELPHIA   ST LOUIS   SYDNEY   TORONTO   2000

CHURCHILL LIVINGSTONE
An imprint of Harcourt Publishers Limited

© Harcourt Publishers Limited 2000

 is a registered trademark of Harcourt Publishers Limited

The right of Stephen Wright and Jean Sayre-Adams to be identified as
authors of this work has been asserted by them in accordance with the
Copyright, Designs and Patents Act 1988

First published 2000

ISBN 0 443 05834 2

British Library of Cataloguing in Publication Data
A catalogue record for this book is available from the British Library.

Library of Congress Cataloging in Publication Data
A catalogue record for this book is available from the Library of Congress.

Note
Medical knowledge is constantly changing. As new information becomes
available, changes in treatment, procedures, equipment and the use of
drugs become necessary. The editors/authors/contributors and the
publishers have, as far as it is possible, taken care to ensure that the
information given in this text is accurate and up to date. However, readers
are strongly advised to confirm that the information, especially with
regard to drug usage, complies with latest legislation and standards of
practice.

The
publisher's
policy is to use
**paper manufactured
from sustainable forests**

Printed in China

Contents

A colour plate section can be found between pages 62–63

Preface

For many years, we have been involved with caring for the carers, especially professionals who have become exhausted and burned out in their work. We have set up retreat and recuperation facilities, and worked in many ways to find the space that would allow carers to let go of the ties that bind them into roles that have come to bring more harm than good. This book is deeply rooted in our experiences down the years, and reinforced by the volume of evidence that is available about the struggles of carers. It is affected also by our own spiritual paths as we have learned to walk our talk – deepening our spiritual practices and learning to be in right relationship, not least with each other.

We are mindful, too, of the separation and disconnectedness that occurs at many levels of society – between professionals and lay carers, among professionals themselves, between organisations and the staff they employ and so on. We notice too how this separation keeps knowledge and practices apart: spirituality is dealt with by religious studies departments, chaplains or the occasional lecture for professionals. And yet, spirituality seems to be everybody's business, it pervades every aspect of our lives whether we are conscious of it or not. Caring also affects every one of us, not just those such as doctors, nurses and other therapists in the healthcare sphere, but lay carers in the home, teachers, social workers, managers, the police, firefighters – every occupation has a caring component to a greater or lesser degree. Often we are unaware of it, yet right relationship could transform the caring context not just in the hospital or nursing home, but in the factory, office and household as well. Thus we believe that so much of what we have sought to present in this book can be applied in countless settings where human beings are together. Meanwhile, many of us seem locked into our own compartments – personal, educational, occupational, social. Isolation, disconnection and distant relationships which do not nourish ourselves or others seem to be the norm.

It is this disconnection that we have sought to address in this book, a separation that keeps people from relating not only to each other, but also to themselves and that which is beyond the self. Without this connection, this right relationship, sacred space cannot reveal itself, and without an awareness of and reverence for the presence of the sacred, the paths of true healing and caring cannot emerge. This book is about pathways towards right relationships for individuals, groups and organisations; restoring wholeness, healing and caring. Waking up to the sacred in health, healing and caring is probably the greatest contribution that we can now make to transform healthcare.

Stephen G. Wright
Jean Sayre-Adams

Cumbria 1999

Acknowledgements

The parts of the text in shaded boxes are vignettes of experience taken from our own and other's stories that we have heard in recent years. We are particularly grateful to Neal Mellon, Ian Turnbull, Cornelia Featherstone, Diane Bright, Bernie Fletcher, Pam Shepherd, Richard Cowling, Chris Johns, Jeanne Achterberg, Frank Lawless, Walter Storey, Diana Dante, Rosy Daniel, David Reilly, Janet Venn, Brenda Mallon, Kate Cicio, Sheila Harvey, Francis Joy, Ann Brimstead, Cliff Panton, Imogen Yates, Fran, Anna and Matthew Jack Biley, Sheila Gilbert, Jeannie Young, Miranda Tufnell, Adam Hill, Geoff Whiteford, Ian Webster, Liz Tipping, Sheila Kendrick, Jo Jones, Djann Hoffman, Lisa Faithorn, Mary and Max Rodel, Robert Preston, Brenda Beck, Jon Weinell, Judith and Russell Rowley, Richard and Gina Farncombe, Annie Hallett, Denise Maxwell, Sandra Bailey, Laura King, Chris Ready, George Lewith, Anne MacDonald, Pat and Christopher Pilkington, David Pilkington, Jane Carr, Clare Rayner, Chris Green, David Lewis, Patrick Barnett, Paul Mayho, Claudio Bardella, Lynne Nicholl, Ann Mills, Mark and Jocelyn Young, Sheila MacDonald and James, John Richmond, Hugh Rooney, Janet Swan, Frances Carol, Frank Ashton, Matthew and Ruth Wright, Jane Salvage, Helen Leathard, Betty Kershaw, Laurence Winram, Janice Little, Susan Todd, Eliza Forder, Rick Steele, Justin and Melanie Bailey, David Bamforth, 'Trevor' and many other friends and colleagues who have given us their contributions, encouragement and support. Special thanks also to John and Eliza Forder, Cindy Pavlinac and Laurence Winram for some of the photographs; and to Inta Ozols, Valerie Dearing and Katrina Mather at Churchill Livingstone for sensitive and loving guidance and support.

For Ram Dass
and
Mother Meera

Introduction

The third millennium will be spiritual or there will be no third millennium'.

Malraux 1995

INTRODUCTION

There is an old story of God and the devil, who were out walking one day. Along the road, they come upon a bright shining object lying in the dirt. God picks it up, holding it up to the sun as it shimmers and shines, and the devil asks: 'What's that?' 'It is the secret of life', replies God. 'Give it to me,' demands the devil, 'I'll organise it!'

In this introduction, we wish to define some of our terms, although we do so with some hesitancy, for to define something can serve to separate it and confine it to a limited perspective rather than to liberate it for creative application and thinking. Indeed, as we will touch upon at several points in this book, the tendency of human beings to organise dogmatically has been the undoing of many a great idea. Our original working title for this book was 'Creating Sacred Space', but the notion of 'creating', to begin with, implies that if we can but put the right components together, be they acts or people or situations or things, then the sacred can be made like a new building on an estate or a new chemical in a laboratory.

If there is a creative act at all, it is one of co-creation, making some difference in ourselves that changes our awareness and shifts our consciousness in some way that brings us to the realisation that sacred space is already here. It has never been away. What has 'been away', if anything, is our own spirit, our own soul, our true self; blindfolded, gagged and earplugged by the personality we inhabit in the world that is so caught up in the drama of everyday things – getting to work, making meals, creating and breaking relationships – that every moment seems to be filled with what we believe to be the only reality. This reality so crowds out every other perspective that we find it difficult, if not impossible most of the time, to be still, to witness, to notice what else is going on. It may be hard to see how well-crafted we have become in acting our part on the stage of life, so that we can no longer see it as anything other than real life. Like a star in a soap opera, playing the part day in and day out, met in the street by 'fans' who call us by the name we play and not our own, interviewed as if the part is the reality and the person beneath is but a fictional irrelevance, we remain stuck in our roles.

Many reports have identified the difficulties of carers, both lay and professional, but the solutions to the various problems are often limited by the narrow view of the role and the needs of the carers. Attention is paid almost exclusively to materialistic issues of support and resources, assuming that all would be well if these could be rectified. While not wishing to diminish the need to work towards such goals, we are sceptical of such a limited perspective. In environments where support and resources are good, carers still struggle to cope, they still burn out, and this implies that something is being overlooked: something in the nature of the caring relationship and what each carer and recipient of care brings to it. It is these relationships that are the focus of this book. Even if a caregiver receives support, such as rest breaks, the emotional labour of caring continues. Our connection, our relationships with the receivers of care can continue to affect us whether we are in their presence or not. Carers care, thus we do certain things and behave in certain ways, fulfilling our prescribed roles. The laws and conventions of the wider world keep us carefully on track in these roles just in case we should decide to deviate. After all, the threat to all the other people involved is potentially enormous. If even one of us, at any one point, were to snap out of it and protest 'Wait a minute, is this how it is really supposed to be? Can't we do it in some other way? Can't we change the plot?', then what might the response be? Probably one of incredulity, mixed with irritation because we are all too busy getting on with it to think about it, spiced with a little fear that if we did stop and take stock, the chasm of possible change that would open before us is too terrifying too contemplate, and anyway we do not have the time, money, staff equipment to do things any differently.

A great many carers, perhaps most as we shall see from the evidence discussed in Chapter 1, are so caught up in doing the caring, playing out the part to the full, that it is almost impossible for us to take a step back for a while and see how our world might be a little different. We are often trapped in difficult roles and circumstances that demand that we give our all (and are drawn into those roles by our own drive to give our all). The roles can ultimately damage the majority of us in all manner of ways. If we perceive any difficulties at all, they are assumed to be readily resolvable if we did but have more money, more staff or more time. Mentioning words like spirituality, sacred and right relationship in such a context is highly problematic. A starving man would argue that his belly needs to be filled first, then if there is time he would be willing to consider the meaning of life later.

We do not deny the need for the correct material resources to meet the demands of caring. There are a great many sources of knowledge and action in the world to pursue this goal, such as the work of large professional or voluntary organisations, lobbying for more staff or money or support, and individual carers who take on the might of the bureaucracies to get what they need. Indeed, both the authors each play very active roles in these arenas to work for better resources and services. However, there is more, as so many of the studies into the struggles of carers have indicated.

Our emphasis in this text is therefore on integration. It is not attention to matters either material or spiritual, but both. Much of the research and debate about the needs of those in caring roles, either lay or professional, has been about resources. We seek to offer an added dimension here that in many respects has been long neglected. We are also suspicious about the linear model that is often presented: demonstrate the need for resources, meet those needs and all will be well. Relationships, holism, the sacred are all very well, but perhaps we will try and fit these in when we are sure that the conditions are right. Our suspicion centres on a wariness of the conditions ever being 'right'. There is no evidence that providing the best of modern pay and working conditions for staff will automatically bring better quality of care and staff satisfaction; there is no evidence that, where the lay carer at home is given all the material resources and support needed, that there is not some deeper dissatisfaction or malaise still at work. Indeed, an added dimension to our suspicions is that, if we pay attention first to right relationship, the sacred and holism, then any system will work better. Getting the relationships right first is the precursor to developing right circumstances and systems, not an add-on luxury that we might consider once the carers have been given the food of the best pay and conditions.

While a focus on money and other resources might seem right and proper, the denial of other factors may be more than a matter of being focused on 'one thing at a time'. 'Once we've got the right numbers of staff available, then we can take a look at these "other things".' However, we suspect that the 'other things' do not get looked at, because 'adequate resources' may be forever out of reach; once one level of need is apparently satisfied, another emerges to take its place. After all, there is no investment, in one sense, in having a totally contented workforce, as most professional and trade union organisations would be wiped out at a stroke. There may be an element of self-justification at work. The portrayal of a continuously demoralised and underpaid workforce (or, in the case of lay carers, their portrayal by voluntary support groups as forever coping inadequately because of poor support) is a necessary component to justify their existence. Furthermore, it may just be that, at some intuitive but unacknowledged level, our focus upon material resources helps us to keep other options at bay: the inner work, the work on relationships, which we may know in our hearts to be the most important, but which perhaps is all a bit too scary. It is our contention, as the evidence in this text unfolds, that the 'other things' are not peripheral, they are core. Being at one with ourselves and those around us is the foundation from which all else emanates.

RIGHT RELATIONSHIP

Becoming at one with ourselves and the wider world may seem, at first hand, a laudable aim. It seems naturally 'better' that people should feel at ease with themselves and others in a complex and often difficult life. But, as we shall see, it is a highly subversive idea. It requires a deep inner journey of exploration, something which many political and religious organisations have sought to prevent through the ages. It shakes us out of the complacency of who we think we are, challenges our view of power structures and institutions and undermines our part in stabilising the status quo. Aware of this, some religious structures have sought to repress any inner exploring, demanding, as Lockhart (1997) has noted, absolute observance to creed and doctrine and labelling any other pathway as the work of Satan. Healthcare workers may find the same mechanism at work in their employing organisations, with their controlling hierarchical structures, power struggles and subtle (and sometimes not so subtle) means of keeping everyone in their place. Caring relatives at home may be faced with the aloof 'I know best' professional and the mighty labour of finding a way through the system when there is a concern or a complaint.

Right relationship dismantles such views of the world and how things should be. Right relationship is not a new idea; it is found in the teachings of many spiritual traditions, both ancient and modern. Right relationship is a harmonious, balanced, attentive, action-orientated way of being in the world. It is built on values of respect and reverence for persons and the whole of creation, seeking to be in relationship with them in patterns which are loving, supportive, available and not hooked on models of power, control and abuse. It seeks to nourish and aid others to choose and pursue their own life path, to make right choices that are equally loving and nourishing for them, without imposing our own will or world-view upon them. Indeed, in right relationship, there is no us and them, no separation, but an acknowledgement of the inescapable interconnectedness of all life, all relationships, all creation. Right relationship requires balanced attention to caring for ourselves as we seek to care for others, and a capacity to let go of old models of helper and helped which keep us stuck in these roles. Thus we are liberated into new patterns of being with people, with the world, which enables us to become aware of the traps of entering prescribed roles with others. Instead, right relationship allows us to let go of being in control of others or of running with fixed agendas about helping and healing, and to rest easily in ourselves and our presence, knowing that our loving, available presence may be all that is needed to allow the other to fulfill his or her own journey towards health and wholeness. In right relationship, we do not so much help others, but become available and centred ourselves in ways which allow the others to help and heal themselves. It is first and foremost about deepening our understanding of ourselves – a slow 'cooking' of the psyche, as James Hillman (1979) suggests. We work to discover who we are, what makes us tick and what has heart and meaning for us; we heal old wounds and we come into a state of being where we can be attentive to the world around us. We seek personal change to be at ease and in harmony with the world and ourselves, and to make ourselves available to work effectively to relieve suffering without harming ourselves.

Such a transformation requires a huge shift in personal consciousness, not least because one of the defences we can often throw up is that 'surely I am conscious anyway?' The shift of consciousness that comes as we enter into right relationship with our deepest selves, our innermost being, utterly transforms our view of the world and our place in it. We 'see through things', understanding better what is real and what is illusion, what is important and what is unimportant. Consciousness of the self has been the key to all sacred traditions, for it is in knowing the self that we go beyond the self, to that place or part of us, that state of being which down the ages has been called the divine, the absolute, God. Clement of Alexandria (in Jung 1979), one of the earliest Christian writers and theologians, noted that 'It is the greatest of all disciplines to know oneself; for when a man knows himself, he knows God'. Yet, paradoxically, this knowing of the self has often been suppressed down through the ages. It is too dangerous to established authority; far better to keep people in their place through rigid adherence to codes and dogmas, be they religious, political or organisational. The excuse is often given that a personal exploration of the self is too dangerous for the individual. Yet, when we know the state we are in, then we can change the state, whether it be ourselves or some aspect of the wider world.

If there is sometimes no apparent investment in, say, an organisation supporting a change of consciousness of its members, there may be inhibitions against such a path inside ourselves. 'Consciousness', as Lockhart (1997) points out, 'by its very nature, has a blind spot – its own almost permanent unconsciousness of that which is supposedly conscious: the self'. Caught up in what the early Gnostic Christians called 'the embrace of Physis' – the limited perception of the world of matter, everyday concerns and bodily needs – it can be very hard to break free and come home to ourselves. Furthermore, the inner knowing that everyone can experience, that 'there must be more', can be repressed because it is all too frightening – far better to stick within the safe remit of this material reality, despite all its pain and suffering, than to take the risky venture into the unknown. The teachings of the Buddha, Jesus, the prophet Mohammed and many other great spiritual leaders all share one thing in common: a focus on the spirit of truth. The spiritual life is thus neither a belief, nor is it experiences allied to beliefs: it is an opening up of the psyche, an introduction of the mind to its own extraordinary dimensions, a bringing into dialogue of the so-called conscious and unconscious minds. The stripping away of differentiation between the two makes available the transcendent experience, the knowledge that we do not end at our skin.

Thus coming to know ourselves, coming into full consciousness, is not merely a psychological experience, a piece of 'personal growth' or fashionable psychotherapy. It is coming to confront:

... one's own depths in silence, when the 'noise of belief' is stilled and the still small voice of a more sensible self has the chance to be heard. There is a voice, but it does not shout slogans or quote biblical texts: it subsumes everything conscious by its density, by its intense and sometimes electric presence. And it is not evoked by wailing prayers or rote prayers or haranguings of the heavens; it is evoked by shutting up, by recollecting (gathering together) the self in silence until all that is scattered and multifarious and disparate and daft comes together in a new and illuminating pattern. (Lockhart 1997).

Without this mindfulness, this re-collecting of the self, any proper human life or spiritual life is impossible. To not be fully conscious is a form of suffering, battered by the winds of everyday reality and our responses to it. To be fully conscious is also a path of suffering, as we shall see in Chapter 5, because of the type of work that is needed. Self-realisation, enlightenment, full consciousness – these are the goals for which countless spiritual teachers through the ages have been our signposts.

Marilyn Ferguson (1994) reminds us that 'The new world that is dancing now like a vision in the night can only be realised by us personally, in our interaction with others. It can't be designed, legislated or ordained by institutions'. Right relationship therefore begins with ourselves. In knowing who we really are, we become whole. It is a resurrection, a waking up from the long sleep of what we thought was the only view of the world. In so doing we affect all around us. When we are in right relationship with ourselves, we are on firm foundation for right relationship with others – patients, clients, loved ones and colleagues. We construct other relationships in and with groups and organisations that embody these same principles, which mirror the balanced person we have become. So often we blame organisations – be they social, political, economic or religious – for all our problems. Yet, the organisations have no life of their own. They are not some disembodied entity, which, if all the people were to withdraw from them would continue as living beings. They reflect those who create them and those who work in them, but that is all. An organisation that is not in right relationship with its workforce, one which rests on models of power, control, punishment, abuse, blaming and shaming, is merely a construct of its creators and participants. We are the participants and the creators at many different levels. Enter right relationship with ourselves, and teams, organisations, families and caring relationships can all enter right relationship too.

CONSCIOUSNESS

Healthcare professionals have often been trained (Dossey et al 1988) to use the term 'state of consciousness' to describe pathological or altered states of consciousness resulting from drug manipulation, metabolic derangement, psychosis, head injury or anoxia. However, into that category must be added the states of daydreaming, dreaming, deep relaxation and meditation.

Consciousness involves left and right hemispheric brain functioning. Barbara Dossey (Dossey et al 1988) suggests that:

... hemispheric differentiation has been oversimplified. Although the left hemisphere is more involved in logical, analytic thought procession and the right is more adept at non logical, non analytical thought processing and spatial tasks, the hemispheres work together at all times. When a person has a hunch or a flash of insight, it is the left hemisphere that processes and synthesises the activities that precede the intuition. An example of the way right and left hemispheres work together occurs when a nurse walks down the hall after leaving a person's bedside and intuitively feels that something is not right. While continuing to walk away from the room, the nurse thinks about objective data, such as no change in physical assessment findings and vital signs within the normal range, but a strong intuitive sense draws the nurse back to the bedside now to see this person in a state of cardiac arrest.

Another way that many people speak of consciousness today invariably refers to the part of the mind that is aware. However, many of the cutting-edge thinkers (and feelers) such as Larry Dossey (1993) believe that we live the 'vast bulk of our psychic lives not in awareness but in unawareness or the unconsciousness. Why do we, when we talk about the place of the mind in health, not consider the unconscious?' He goes on to suggest that perhaps it is because we 'don't trust the unconscious. Many people see it as a sinister force that pushes them around against their will ... a dark repository of unacceptable, unflattering thoughts and emotions such as lust, hatred, and greed. Freud, who believed that the unconscious could not be trusted, was largely responsible for this'. The Freudian view maintains that the unconscious is the 'region of the id, a domain of psychic force compelling us, among other things, to hate our mother or father, to have incestuous desires and homicidal thoughts, and to indulge in unacceptable fantasies and wishes' (Dossey 1993). The Jungian view, however, sees the unconscious quite differently, as the 'home of timeless psychic forces he called archetypes, which generally are invariant throughout all cultures and eras, He felt that every psychic force has its opposite in the unconscious – the force of light is always counterpoised with that of darkness, good with evil, life with death, on and on ... and that any psychic energy could get out of hand and things become unbalanced ... that human beings could have "too much harmony and goodness"' (Dossey 1993). In order to be whole we need to integrate the darker parts of ourselves with the light – the unconscious with the conscious. Expanding on this theme, we believe the unconscious parts of ourselves are endless; there are so many dimensions of ourselves of which we are unaware. Coming into health or wholeness happens only as we open to these dimensions. Indeed, Newman (1986) theorises that true health is possible only if our consciousness continues to expand – that disease (dis-ease) presents itself, whether of body, mind or spirit, when we block this expansion. Newman also suggests that dis-ease of any kind is the way our innate consciousness alerts us to the places where we are stuck.

As we attempt to contemplate the awesomeness of what the full potential of consciousness implies, we come to know that we are not alone. Consciousness is eternal and infinite; it is impossible for us comprehend it all in conventional terms. Some of our ancestors spoke of 'universal mind' and tended to have an unbounded view of consciousness that had important spiritual implications. Mystical and spiritual texts down the ages affirm this view. More than 2000 years ago, for example, Hermes Trismegistus said:

Make yourself grow to a greatness beyond measure, by a bound free yourself from the body: raise yourself above all time, become Eternity: then you will understand God. Believe that nothing is impossible for you, think yourself immortal and capable of understanding all, all arts, all sciences, the nature of every living being. Mount higher than the highest height: descend lower than the lowest depth. Draw into yourself all sensation of everything created, fire and water, dry and moist, imagining that you are everywhere, on earth, in the sea, in the sky, that you are not yet born, in the maternal womb, adolescent, old, dead, beyond earth. If you embrace in your thought all things at once, times, places, substances, qualities, quantities, you may understand God. (Copenhaver 1992).

Pert (1997) says, with reverence, 'God is a molecule'.

ENERGY

The idea of 'energy' or 'subtle energy' that is continuously used in alternative/complementary therapies is one that comes under a great deal of criticism. Scores of different words and concepts across many cultures are used to describe 'energy', and they are often used interchangeably in a mix-and-match way in much of 'New Age' thinking. The Chinese refer to *ch'i*, in India we find *prana*, among the Jews it is *nefish* – all are labels for the energy that practitioners say they work with that precipitates healing. Some of the most fascinating work on the understanding of energy is being done by Dr Valerie Hunt, a Professor at the University of California, Los Angeles. Dossey (1997), however, warns us that perhaps we are being too limited in our comprehension of energy; the terms adored by a variety of complementary therapists as an invariable part of the natural order may have been invented, and it is possible that 'healing' is much greater than we can yet comprehend. Modern science only recognises four forms of energy: gravity, strong and weak nuclear forces and electromagnetic. Much of the jargon in the field of healing, complementary therapies and general 'New Age' speak applies the term 'energy' to all manner of healing approaches, yet is unable to measure or define its nature. While there may well be other forms of subtle energy at work, we need to be cautious about laying claims that cannot be substantiated. To do so exposes us to ridicule from the scientific establishment, and can make it difficult to advance complementary and other healing perspectives in the orthodox, scientifically dominated healthcare world.

Consciousness and energy are greater than our five senses can perceive, and in these areas, there is much that has only been revealed using approaches that stand outside conventional acceptance, such as mystical experiences. Karl Pribram (Talbot 1991) believes that there may be all kinds of things that our brains have learned to edit out of our visual reality, such as transcendental experiences or (in the case of Therapeutic Touch practitioners) the seeing or feeling of human energy fields.

However, Dossey (1997) believes that it may only be justifiable to use the concept of 'energy' in a provisional, qualified, metaphorical way; that to use it as a concrete reality may blind us to the true nature of healing. He goes on to warn that to present something as scientifically proven when it is not, can be disastrous. Dossey tells the story of the restaurant in the Ozark Mountains of northern Arkansas where one day they introduced a new item on the menu – beef stroganoff. It was a resounding failure: no one would order it. The next day the owner changed the name to beef and noodles. It was an immediate success and became the most popular item on the menu. Dossey suggests therefore that the moral of the story is 'if you want to sell it, be careful what you call it'. When we use the term 'energy' in this book, we use it in the way it is being used currently in the alternative/complementary literature, but with the understanding that we may be using it metaphorically.

HOLISM

There is a tendency among carers to use the word 'holism' in reference to the body–mind–spirit, and to imply that they are practising holism if they administer a bed bath and give medications (body), refer the patient to a psychotherapist or social worker to sort out their problems (mind), and ask about the patient's religious preference and call a vicar, priest or minister (spirit). When we use the concept of holism in this book, it is in quite a different context.

A new paradigm (a map or blueprint of reality) is emerging in all disciplines. In healthcare, this is a paradigm that is moving away from the Newtonian pragmatists where everything is seen as mechanistic and reductionist (viewing the person as essentially a group of body systems interacting in predictable ways) to a new perspective of an interconnected universe as envisioned by post-Einsteinian thinkers. This thinking encourages a more holistic view of people – not just an interrelationship of 'biopsychospiritual' factors, but seeing each human being as part of the universe which is a dynamic web of interconnected and interrelated events, none of which function in isolation. Bohm (1973), a protégé of Einstein's and one of the world's most respected quantum physicists, wrote:

There has been too little emphasis on what is, in our view, the most fundamentally different new feature of all, i.e. the intimate interconnectedness of different systems that are not in spatial contact … the parts are seen to be in immediate connection, in which their dynamical relationships depend, in an irreducible way, on the state of the whole system (and indeed on that broader system in which they are contained, extending ultimately and in principle to the entire universe). Thus one is led to a new notion of unbroken wholeness which denies the classical idea of analysability of the world into separately and independently existent parts.

Each of us as human beings is a part of this whole; each has a unique part to play, and furthermore, the whole cannot be whole without our unique participation within it.

Other scientists beside Bohm take a similar view. For instance, Pribram, a neurophysiologist at Stanford University indicates that the universe itself is a kind of giant hologram, a three-dimensional picture that contains all things. He and scientists like him suggest that there is evidence that our world and everything in it are projections from a level of reality beyond time and space. Embracing this holographic model helps to explain virtually all paranormal and mystical experiences (Talbot 1991). In addition, it is thought that each individual cell within our body is a hologram and contains within it everything that ever was or ever will be. If this mind-blowing concept is anywhere near the truth, and the truth is something probably even greater, we contain within our consciousness the possibility to embody the knowledge and wisdom of all time!

Although many of these ideas are extremely controversial and not yet accepted by a majority of scientists, many important and distinguished thinkers do support them and believe that they might form the most accurate picture of reality that we have to date. Science appears to be moving by deduction to the same view that mystics and metaphysical poets have reached by induction – that everything is connected, and the greatest is also to be found in the smallest:

> To see a World in a Grain of Sand
> And a Heaven in a Wild Flower,
> Hold Infinity in the palm of your hand
> And Eternity in an hour.

William Blake

Moving away from the elation of what may be and grounding the definition of holism into a working one for purposes of this book, we are inclined towards Dossey et al's (1988) perspective: 'Holism is the view that an integrated whole has a reality independent of and greater than the sum of its parts'.

SACRED SPACE

Coming into right relationship is a sacred act. Entering the place of stillness in ourselves, set apart momentarily from what we come to realise are the trivia of life where we can discover our true being, indeed just 'be', we can re-connect with our senses and return to the world to participate fully and safely in all its beauty and tragedy. Making time for stillness helps us to come home to ourselves, and discover that home is sacred. This has been the focus of spiritual teachings for millennia. The word 'sacred' has its origins in the Latin *sacrare*: to consecrate or make holy. It is deeply imbued with religious and spiritual connotations, concerning rituals and practices associated with our desire to understand and connect with the divine such as sacred music or writings. The Bible, the Qur'an and the Upanishads are sacred texts. Much of the finest music, prose and poetry across the generations has been inspired by and has sought to represent the sacred. Sacred space, and its instruments – beauty, stillness, music and so on – inspires and uplifts us. It 'fills us with awe, with joy, with wellbeing, that which adds meaning to our lives' (Angwin 1998). The sacred concerns reverence for all of life, for rituals and places that connect us to that deep core in our being that we have called the Self, God, the Absolute, the One. Sacred space can be places where we feel that connection more strongly than in others, where there is 'a construction in the imagination that affirms the independence of the holy' (Lane 1988). Sacred space is the instrument of our unfolding spirituality, the tool to do the work; it is also the realised outcome as we discover the sacred in all things, including ourselves.

Can we 'make' sacred space? It is possible to set up an altar in our office, build a shrine in our garden or create a certain ceremony or ritual, but these do not become sacred in themselves. Things become sacred because of the significance and reverence with which we hold them. They form part of a sacred act because of the consciousness from ourselves with which we imbue them, the beliefs and feelings we attach to them. As we shall see in the discussion in Chapter 4, there are innumerable pathways to the sacred. The sacred can therefore be 'out there' in terms of special places or actions: a religious service, a particularly beautiful forest or landscape, a special building or site. While there are many places that 'feel' different, because of their inherent structure or presence of earth energies, it may be that they are just places where we are more aware of the sacred. Places that are timeless, where we nourish our souls, re-connect with the world, re-collect ourselves. Places where the environment outside matches the geography within, our particular path or state of being at the time. Places where we can alter our perceptions of reality and integrate this knowledge into new patterns of self-knowledge for being in the world.

To 'create' sacred space is thus, for us, a contradiction in terms. If everything is part of the whole and interconnected, then everything is sacred. All that changes is our awareness of it. Thus we do not so much 'make' sacred space, insofar as we may change the physical environment in some way, as recognise it and participate in it by shifting our awareness toward the sacred. Sacred space is both internal and external, within us and beyond, it is 'here' already, eternally present, all we have to do is 'tune in' to it, become aware of it, realise it. The sacred is all around us and in each one of us: we do not so much create sacred space as co-create with it, come to an awareness of it, know it, pay attention to it and participate mindfully in it (Fig. I. 1). Emerson (Bode 1981) writes that when a man's 'mind is illuminated, and his heart is kind, he throws himself joyfully into the sublime order, and does, with knowledge, what the stones do by structure'.

Sacred space is a place where wonder can be revealed, where the 'divine or the supernatural can be glimpsed or experienced, where we can get in touch

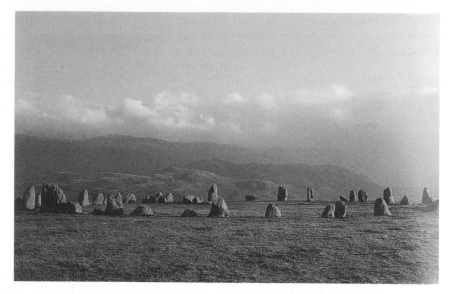

Figure I.1 People have marked certain places as sacred for millenia: the ancient stone circle at Castelrigg, Cumbria. © Forder & Forder, reprinted with permission.

with that which is larger than ourselves' (Streep 1997). Getting in touch with sacred space requires active intention, using pathways to discover it, such as those we suggest in Chapter 4. Having become aware of its possibility, it then allows us to work with it, to enhance healing environments, to have respect for all that is taking place in our immediate world and the wider world around us. In opening to the sacred, the intention is to move beyond reverence into compassionate action. Sacred space is a place of spiritual work, where the consciousness and power of ourselves and the universe engage in a wondrous interplay that seeks to set all around it in right relationship, to re-collect into wholeness and thereby heal (Plate 1).

In this book, we have allied the concept of sacred space to the work of healers and carers, whoever and wherever they may be, because we believe that every healing and caring act is a sacred act. In the work world of most carers, replete with myriad distractions and pressures, the sense of the sacred has been almost completely lost. A few hardy souls may have the strength to integrate it quietly into their work, but for most, if the sacred or spirituality are mentioned at all, they are the subject of scepticism, ridicule or embarrassment. Caught in the struggle of doing the day-to-day work, we find it hard to stand back from it and take a wider view. Healing and caring still happen, but in ways that are stunted, their potential unfulfilled because right relationships in all parts of the caring context are not fully present. We believe that a restoration and renewal of the sacred in healing and caring work is both timely and essential, for the good of our interpersonal relationships, for the good of the organisations that seek to provide care, and for the good of the planet. Sacred space does not end at the doors of the sick person's bedroom, the clinic or nursing home, or the hospital ward. It pervades everything, and is available to us in all places and at all times.

In Chapter 4, we will look at how a sense of the sacred is nourished by qualities of certain places. It is this 'spirit of place', or rather the loss of it, that affects right relationship in all manner of ways. Referring to the work of ancient peoples who constructed the great tombs and stone circles of neolithic times, Palmer & Palmer (1997) write:

Sacred, sacrosanct, sanctuary
In the ruins of what was sacred space that we need back:

These monoliths to moon and sun remind us
That we abandoned the stars for ourselves, only to find
That we have no rite for being human

But now as the breeze stirs, we slow our steps
Where stone breathes we can receive its whispered gift again.

In this book, we will look at ways we can both receive this 'whispered gift again' and create 'rites for being human' through right relationship.

Henry Miller (cited in McLuhan 1996) believes that 'our destination is never a place, but rather a new way of looking at things'. The potential of the sacred is enhanced when we wake up to it, when we seek to work with it and hold it in our everyday lives. Its power is unleashed when we seek to create certain spaces that shift our consciousness to the presence of the sacred. It is made fully manifest when we are spurred to action in the world, not in the narrow confines of our own goals and ambitions, but being available as conscious participants, playmates of the sacred, aiding its full realisation in every caring moment, every action, no matter how mundane or profound. When we are in right relationship with ourselves, the effects ricochet down and out into all our relationships. When we are in right relationship with ourselves, we discover the sacred space that is within. In that discovery comes the realisation that what is within is also beyond us – as above, so below. Attuning to the sacred within, we find it in everything as well. Thus grounded and centred in our own being, our own sacredness, we become available for the sacred to radiate into all aspects of our lives, not least our caring and healing work. Thus, we do not so much create sacred space, as become and be it. Who we are is the sacred. Who we are is the healer.

REFERENCES

Angwin R 1998 Creating sacred space. Positive Health Dec/Jan: 6–7
Bode C 1981 The portable Emerson. Viking, New York
Bohm D 1973 Quantum theory as an indication of a new order in physics; implicate and explicate order in physical law. Foundation of Physics 3:139–168
Copenhaver B 1992 Hemetica. Cambridge University Press, Cambridge
Dossey B, Keegan L, Guzzetta C, Kolkmeier L 1988 Holistic nursing – a handbook for practice. Aspen, Gaithersburg

Dossey L 1993 Healing words. Harper, San Francisco

Dossey L 1997 The forces of healing; reflections on energy, consciousness and the beef stroganoff principle. Alternative Therapies in Health and Medicine 3(5):8–14

Ferguson M 1994 Aquarius now – making it through the confusion gap. Catalist. Nov/Dec: 34–47

Hillman J 1979 The dream of the underworld. Harper & Row, New York

Jung C G 1979 (Hull R F trans). Aion: researches into the phenomenology of self. Princeton, New York

Lane B C 1988 Landscapes of the sacred. Paulist, New York

Lockhart D 1997 Jesus – the heretic. Element, Shaftesbury

Malraux A 1995 cited in the Temple of Understanding Newsletter. Spring

McLuhan T C 1996 Cathedrals of the spirit. Thorsons, London

Newman M 1986 Health as expanding consciousness. Mosby, St Louis

Palmer M, Palmer N 1997 Sacred Britain. Piatkus, London

Pert C 1997 Molecules of emotion. Scribner, New York

Streep P 1997 Altars made easy. Harper Collins, London

Talbot M 1991 The holographic universe. HarperCollins, New York

1

Caring can make you sick

'Prisoner, tell me, who was it that bound you?'
'It was my master,' said the prisoner. 'I thought I could outdo
everybody in the world in wealth and power, and I amassed in my
own treasure-house the money due to my king. When sleep
overcame me I lay upon the bed that was for my lord, and on
waking up I found I was a prisoner in my own treasure house.'
'Prisoner, tell me who was it that wrought this unbreakable chain?'
'It was I,' said the prisoner, 'who forged this chain very carefully. I
thought my invincible power would hold the world captive leaving
me in a freedom undisturbed. Thus night and day I worked at the
chain with huge fires and cruel hard strokes. When at last the work
was done and the links were complete and unbreakable, I found
that it held me in its grip.'

Rabindranath Tagore, Gitanjali

Psychotics know that two and two come to five.
Co-dependents know that two and two are four – but they can't
stand it!

Anon.

THE TIES THAT BIND

In any caring relationship, whether between professional carer and patient
or between friends or family members, we are exposed to a huge range of
questions and concerns. The traditional image of the self-sacrificing,
dedicated, heroic doctor, nurse, partner, friend or relative, giving all for the
good of another is burned deep into our consciousness. That's the way it
should be if we are to be good, that's the way we are bound in the carer –
cared-for relationship. The carer gives, the patient receives.

Such a view is far too limiting in its scope. It ignores the trend towards more
holistic ways of working between caregivers and care receivers. It leaves out
the interconnectedness of the two – for in reality, both give and receive. It
omits the energy and support needed by the carer in order to keep on caring.
By and large, carers are expected to cope with caring, and if they can't, then
the chances are that others will assume a weakness on the part of the carer
rather than a lack of help or resources. The carer is expected to perform
altruistically, with caring itself frequently being seen as sufficient reward for
the work done. And so professional carers have often found themselves low
down on national pay scales – financial rewards are assumed to be of

secondary importance. In the home, the informal carer is often bound by a sense of familial duty or expectation that he or she will take on the caring role for a family member or friend when the need arises. This is all the more so when there is a strong bond of love for the one who needs care. For the professional carer, there are often bonds of love too. Not the personal, intimate loving relationship that exists, say, between mother and child or between partners, but a form of love all the same. Huge numbers of healthcare workers report that what motivated them to join their professions was a desire to help others, to work with people, to express a need to care for others. James Hillman (cited in Campbell 1984) notes that 'Just as he who comes to me needs me for help, so I need him to express my need to give help'.

'Agape', love for another that is not bound by personal or sexual desires or attachments, underpins much of the work of the professional carer. Alastair Campbell (1984) sees this as a form of 'moderated love', as an appropriate connection between carer and cared-for. Such an approach permits caring concern and action for the other, but also permits a certain distance which prevents the carers becoming so involved that they become exhausted or burned out. Challenging the notion of altruism, Campbell, like Hillman, also suggests that caring relationships are far more complex than an apparently simple, linear process where the carers simply give to others without thought for themselves. When we care for another, whether we acknowledge it or not, it is likely that we are fulfilling a need – to be needed, for power over the other, to keep the other alive to avoid the pain of loss – that is as important as what we give.

> When my mother was dying, I gave up work to take care of her. I never gave it a second thought. I loved her and would do anything for her. I would cry myself to sleep every night as she slowly faded away. I wept with frustration at my inability to control her pain, to make her understand me or to get the doctors and nurses to do what I knew was best for her. It never occurred to me not to make the sacrifice, she was my mother, of course I must be the one to take care of her, I couldn't possibly see her spend her last days in a home or a hospice, she would have wanted to die in her own bed, and I felt it was up to me to make sure that happened. I don't think I could have lived with myself afterwards had I not done everything myself for her in her last days.

The struggle to care for someone who is close to us and whom we love will inevitably bring pain and suffering to ourselves. Our love for others (whatever form this takes), our own needs and motivations, our personal and social expectations about duty to care – all these can bind us into relationships where caring for others tests the limits of our self-awareness, our coping strategies, our innermost drives and incentives. Often we may be unaware of these until something 'cracks'. In pouring our energies into meeting the needs of others, we may find ourselves emotionally, physically and spiritually drained, acting out our roles in the great drama of pain and suffering without thought or consequence for ourselves. Attached, willingly or unwillingly, to our part in the play, 'doing' compassion as hard as we can, we may find it impossible to stand back and let go of the ties that bind us into caring. Many people deal with such events in their lives with equanimity, loving the other while simultaneously knowing and setting their own boundaries and taking care of themselves. Many others, however, do not.

DYING TO TAKE CARE OF YOU

An increasing body of evidence points to the intensity of the labour involved in caring, and the impact it has on the carer. Whether lay or professional, it seems that the potential for suffering among carers is enormous. When a person reaches a state of physical, emotional or mental exhaustion, burnout occurs, and it appears to affect both lay and professional carers alike. Almberg's study, for example, suggests that exhaustion and burnout from caring happen in many different cultures and that 'relatives who have been giving care for many years may experience similar emotional exhaustion to that suffered by staff' (Almberg et al 1997). Whether lay carers would express their state as burnout is questionable, since it tends to be a term mostly used in professional discussion, but there is evidence of high levels of stress and illness among informal or lay carers (e.g. Henwood 1998). Lay carers, in one study (Princess Royal Trust 1998), felt that it was not even of interest to professional carers whether they could cope or not. Over 70% of 1300 lay carers involved in this study reported that it was largely assumed that they would cope with looking after a person at home, and were not asked if they could do so. Are they not being asked because of ignorance, because of fears of what might turn up if they were asked, because of denial ... what is not known about does not hurt? Professional carers, however, are supposed to have special training which equips them to deal with the suffering of others dispassionately, maintaining a certain distance which 'protects' both them and their patients or clients.

It was drilled into me as a student nurse, 'You must never get involved!' Sitting on a patient's bed to offer comfort while he was dying you would be told 'Have you no work to do?' The whole ethos of my professional preparation was that I must keep separate from patients, that I must never show my feelings. That patients expect me to be kind and efficient, but somehow remote and disinterested. That I should behave like this, it was argued, was in the best interests of myself and the patients. They expect us to be cool and aloof so that we could deal with all their problems objectively. We must behave this way so that we do not get upset by their pain and difficulties. That way, it was argued, we would be able to cope, to sleep at night with untroubled minds, to get on with the work without it being troubled by disruptive emotions. It took me 20 years to realise what a load of nonsense this all was. The whole of my profession seemed to be caught up in a sort of collective delusion that it was possible to work this way. I and my colleagues probably spent more time and energy trying to bottle up or hide our feelings than we did actually having them. What a farce, a whole caring profession built on the edifice of actually denying caring. And it was the same for everyone I met – policemen, social workers, firemen, doctors, ambulance men – it was all the same story. Keep a distance. Don't show your feelings. Little did I know the price I paid when I bought into this contract … Don't get involved. How utterly stupid! How can you care and not be involved? It's true that we have to cope. It's true that we can't afford to fall apart when the people we are caring for may be doing just that. But there had to be a better way. Why couldn't someone have taught us how to manage feelings instead of trying to bury them? Why couldn't someone have taught us about limits and boundaries and involvement and managing relationships instead of trying to maintain this enormous, wasteful illusion?

Salvage (1985) writing from a nursing context and Dossey (1995) from a medical viewpoint both suggest that fostering the internalisation of feelings, as part of the socialisation of healthcare workers, has serious consequences for the carer. Doctors, nurses and others, including perhaps lay carers, are all given clear signals that we are supposed to act as if 'we can take it': don't complain, never ask for help, never call for more resources, no matter how difficult the situation becomes. If we break this unwritten rule, the response of the uncaring culture is often to blame the victim. The carer who complains may find themselves being asked 'What is wrong with you that makes you unable to cope?' instead of getting a response that recognizes that more help is needed. The impact of this attitude, this whole cultural approach to caring, is chilling.

Evidence is accumulating about the price that is paid by carers, both lay and professional. The World Health Organization (WHO) (1994) saw burnout, the exhaustion and loss of function associated with stress at work, as a major problem for healthcare professionals. Factors such as inadequate resources, lack of involvement in decision-making at work, authoritarian leadership styles, excessive case loads and poor staff relationships are all cited as significant causes. Similar factors appear in a Health Education Authority report (1996), which noted the principal effects of stress as emotional symptoms (e.g. depression, hopelessness, despair, anger, frustration, reduced enjoyment at work and home, suicidal feelings), behavioural changes (e.g. poor concentration and decision-making, absenteeism, marital and work conflicts, increased use of tobacco and alcohol and physical effects (e.g. high levels of various illnesses such as infections, back pain and headaches. The report also highlighted a number of causes specific to the health services. Like the WHO report, it found the causes of stress to lie in heavy workloads and lack of support, but emphasised also:

- ineffective communication and consultation systems
- invasion of personal space and lack of respect for functional and professional boundaries
- pressures leading to an inappropriate management style
- loss of support in a work community through radical reorganisation
- financial considerations taking precedence over human resource considerations, and the problem of getting the right balance between the two

- disputes between managers and medical consultants, and between other groups of staff
- lack of coordination between departments and between individuals
- patients and families being more demanding following the Patient's Charter
- threats of physical and verbal abuse
- exclusion from consultation on policy-making until after key decisions have been made
- work overload through lack of control of patient admissions and accelerated throughput from the reduction of waiting lists
- excessive paperwork – performance statistics that are quantitative and not qualitative
- performance measures that distort decision-making
- lack of trust between managers and staff and between disciplines
- pressure on acute services, because of social services policies and practices
- contracts negotiated without consultation with those who will be involved in fulfilling them
- bringing together different organisational cultures as a consequence of change.

There seems little doubt that many of the above points are coloured by specific changes in the UK National Health Service (NHS) over the past 20 years. During that time, enormous changes have taken place in workplace practices. Not coincidentally, large numbers of workers have left to take early retirement on sickness grounds or to start careers in independent practice. Many of the latter seem to have found their way as independent complementary therapy practitioners. Others have sought to learn such practices and integrate them into their work as a means of producing more holistic caring and better team relationships.

An organisational culture that does not nourish and care for its staff often demonstrates the same symptoms of stress that appear in the staff themselves: an inability to function effectively, grasping at short-term or quick-fix solutions in an effort to resolve or hide the problem, blaming the victim rather than dealing with the cause. (Perhaps this also applies to societies in which individual members feel alienated or unsupported when caring for others at home.) In turn, if the organisation is sick, then the staff who identify with it may take on the same characteristics. 'We attach to the organisation (held in the mind) the same emotions so that, to a greater or lesser degree, the members of the organisation will experience the same feelings as a result of their inter-relatedness with the holding environment' (Stapley 1996). In such settings, staff themselves will respond in a wide variety of ways.

Feeling helpless at work, we may resort to blaming everyone and everything around us for problems, perhaps internalising this and blaming ourselves as well, especially when things go wrong and a patient or client suffers. Blaming is often a sign that we feel helpless in a situation (Stapley 1996), and it is closely related to another classic victim response – the whinge. Maya Angelou (1994) has a warning to offer us about this: 'So watch yourself about complaining, sister. If you can't change a thing, change the way you think about it. Whining is not only graceless, but dangerous. It can alert a brute that a victim is in the neighbourhood.' Whining when we feel helpless is unlikely to produce a positive reaction from the manager, who is probably equally hard-pressed and caught up in the sickness of the organisation. Whingeing and whining are simply expressions of blaming the other for our problems. We try to justify our own status, self-esteem and effectiveness, to preserve some good feelings about ourselves in the face of a sick, often hostile, context. Nevertheless, whingeing is not the response of someone often labelled the 'negative personality' who always has something to complain about, it is a cry of pain in the face of helpless feelings and a hopeless organisation.

Whingeing and victim-blaming are serious problems for any individual or organisation, yet the difficulties go even deeper. Carers in organisations such as hospitals or community teams tend to blame the organisation, while lay carers at home see the problem lying with the social services providers, or government, or society as a whole. In the face of helplessness, wherever we define the organisation to be, the sickness can be found 'out there'. It seems we find it very difficult to look clearly at what is going on around us, to look objectively and without attachment at the sources of our difficulties. After all, if a particular organisation is sick, and you're part of that organisation, and that organisation is part of society, then where does the 'blame' or the 'fault' originate? If only we had more money, staff, resources, nicer bosses, or whatever, then these would solve all our problems. With shoulders to the wheel and noses to the grindstone, we are in a very difficult position from which to look up and see how the world might be different. A cycle of victim behaviour and blaming can come to characterise our every action, and for many, the personal consequences can be very serious indeed.

A study published by the Nuffield Trust (Williams et al 1998) highlighted what had long been a subject of interest in the healthcare media: the levels of stress, sickness, absenteeism and burnout among professional carers. This report, from an authoritative and reputable organisation, brought together much of the prevailing evidence about the alarming state of the NHS workforce, which, despite a growing independent sector, is still responsible for giving over 90% of health care in the UK. The report states that 'for the sake of good management and from simple compassion, both we and the Government should view these findings with due alarm, and accept shared responsibility for working quickly together to develop a programme for action.

Studies highlighting stress and burnout in professional carers continue to mount. Kapur et al (1998) demonstrated continuing high levels of stress among consultants and junior doctors, and a report by Sarah Boseley (1998) raised further alarms about stress among medical staff and the connection with high levels of drug and alcohol abuse. The Professions Allied to Medicine (1998), which includes radiographers, chiropodists, physiotherapists and dieticians, have also recently reported exceptional low morale and high stress levels among a survey of 1800 members. A further report from the University of Sheffield (Borril et al 1998) took account of the views of 11 000 NHS staff. More than one-quarter were suffering from significant levels of stress, with nurses being 40% more likely to suffer stress than other groups of technical and professional workers with whom they were compared.

Other reports in the past which have highlighted similar problems have often been quietly sidelined, not just because they were dismissed as the product of whingeing professionals, but because of fears about public alarm. The Nuffield Trust findings might indeed seem alarming. Over 170 previous research reports are cited in support of the findings, and evidence of attempts to deal with the problems is included. Once again we find such issues as workload pressures, job insecurity, interpersonal conflicts and lack of support topping the list of the causes of the problems. The end result is that 21–50% of doctors show high levels of psychological disturbance, ranging from anxiety through emotional exhaustion to clinical depression and suicide. Similar figures are found among nurses, managers, the professions allied to medicine such as physiotherapists and speech therapists, dentists, pharmacists and ambulance personnel. For all groups, the levels of distress are significantly higher than in equivalent occupations outside the health services. (Interestingly, where similar stresses occur in the non-NHS workforce, similar effects on staff are reported.)

So, on top of professional attitudes which require carers to remain aloof, pressures of work lead huge numbers of carers to succumb to all manner of ills and disconnection from their work and each other. Stress piles upon stress until something has to give – usually the carer has some form of health crisis, or simply 'switches off'. The very people we once sought to care for may become our problem and some healthcare workers respond to this by becoming increasingly remote and impersonal. At a wider level, there are other costs of all this pain to the workforce. Relationships outside work also suffer as the difficulties at work are transmitted to the home. Lay carers experience a similar phenomenon outside the immediate caring relationship (Mazhindu 1998). The costs in financial terms are enormous – one survey by the Confederation of British Industry in 1991 put the loss to employers nationally caused by staff sickness due to stress at over £5 bn. A 1998 Audit Commission report suggested that each NHS trust loss £1.5 m annually because of excessively high staff turnover. A new factor is increasingly entering the cost equation – that of compensation claims by staff. Those who suffer the ill-effects of stress at work are now more likely to receive sympathetic hearings by the courts. A landmark decision in 1998 sent shock waves through many healthcare employers: an NHS trust was ordered to pay substantial damages to the widow of an employee after her husband, suffering from workplace-induced stress, committed suicide. Fears of litigation are helping to focus the minds of those with responsibility for stress at work (Griffiths et al 1995).

CARING FOR THE CARERS

As awareness of the effects of stress upon carers has grown, an increasing number of steps have been taken to counter the problem. Lay carers may find that there is access to respite or counselling facilities to aid them in their work, and many voluntary associations offer help through mutual support groups. Organisations have tried to introduce measures which give more direct support to the staff and produce more staff-friendly managerial cultures. Other organisations and consulting agencies have been set up to research and advise on stress management. Books and papers on the subject fill the library shelves and occupy the attentions of countless programme planners and educators. A scan through the literature suggests that a huge range of options have been attempted. These include:

- policies to involve staff more in decisions at work
- introducing staff counselling services
- improving pay and conditions of service
- monitoring workloads and reducing them where excessive
- teaching stress management, assertiveness and relaxation skills
- introducing exercise and healthy eating programmes
- access to occupational health services
- better training in interpersonal skills
- developing and implementing anti-bullying and anti-discrimination policies at work
- introducing personal development plans
- developing clinical supervision and debriefing groups among staff to provide professional support
- introducing family-friendly policies (e.g. opportunities for career breaks, job sharing, flexible hours, crèche facilities)
- taking steps to reduce violence in the workplace
- giving staff more control over their own work
- developing stress management groups
- developing 'listening groups' (teams of staff who collect information about staff experiences to identify causes of stress and make recommendations)
- team building
- opportunities for time out
- access to continuing education and better job-related training
- better careers counselling.

All of these and more have been implemented with varying degrees of success in a wide variety of organisations. Attempts to help staff feel valued and cared for are legion, and each can contribute to making the carer's workplace or home a more supportive place. An incremental approach, where the more options that are in place, the better the possible outcomes, would seem to be logical. However, it is not our intention in this book to discuss all these approaches in detail. Each has its part to play and we would not wish to question the usefulness of any of them. Some aspects will be taken up in greater detail in Chapter 3, but our concern here is to illuminate the extent of the problem and some of the underlying causes.

The solutions often run the risk of 'fire fighting' – dealing with the problem after it has arisen rather than preventing it in the first place. Doing the latter requires a wholesale commitment to examine and change the organisational culture, the way in which people work together, and the ways that individuals participate in that culture. While it is important to examine workplace conditions and organisational systems and cultures, and to effect changes that may help staff to cope with stress and make the workplace a better place to be, there are other issues operating. The evidence cited so far tends to skirt around these. What are these issues? We get some clues from the common concern of carers that relationships are not working – relationships with employers, with work colleagues, with patients – that something doesn't seem right. The 'something' appears to be not just decent rates of pay, stress reduction techniques or better working conditions – laudable as it is to address such matters. Even when these issues are rectified, the problems seem to persist. Something more is amiss, and it is the 'something more' that this book will seek to explore.

Some hints as to the deeper nature of the problem can be found. Dossey (1995), for example, argues that 'At the root of the problem lies the fact that we, as a culture, have turned our collective back on healing … ignoring the role of consciousness, soul, spirit, and meaning – stock items in the arsenal of authentic healers – we have birthed a malaise that permeates not just the healing profession, but our entire society'. Can it be that the alarming list of difficulties so far discussed that many carers face is only part of the story? Can it be that other factors are at work which seek to undermine effective caring relationships? If the answer to both of these questions is 'yes', then we need to examine what is going on in the caring relationship in a little more detail. Workloads and working conditions undoubtedly have a part to play in causing stress in caring, yet there are other factors too. It is worth noting that problems with relationships are often mentioned as a stress factor, and attempts to deal with these include team-building work. Perhaps there are other areas where the quality of a relationship is having an impact upon a carer's performance. As we seek to change the system and its culture we have to remember that these are not disembodied entities with a life of their own 'out there': we are the culture, we are the system. Who we are, each and every one of us, counts – each of us brings our own particular building block to add to the whole.

THINGS FALL APART

Caring relationships, as we suggested at the beginning of this chapter, are not a linear process from carer to cared for. Both parties and all those involved bring their own scripts into the greater drama. Frank (1991) notes that:

'When the caregiver communicates to the ill person that she cares about their uniqueness, she makes their life meaningful and as that person's life story becomes part of her own, the caregiver's life is made meaningful as well. Care is inseparable from understanding, and like understanding, it must be symmetrical. Listening to another, we hear ourselves. Caring for another, we either care for ourselves, as well, or we end in burnout and frustration.'

The interconnectedness of the caring relationship means that we cannot ignore the part each of us brings into it. If we are struggling to care, it becomes that much more difficult to acknowledge the other's uniqueness. Weighed down by difficult caring contexts and by the possibility that something in each of us finds it difficult to connect with others, we may end up shutting ourselves off from those around us. Perhaps this is a factor in the escalating levels of complaints about professional carers by the public. Caught up in our helper–helped roles we may 'just miss' (Ram Dass & Gorman 1990) fully connecting with the other's suffering, in part because of busy workloads and difficult caring situations, but in part also because we are trapped by the limitations of professional caring relationships and the fear that we may not be able to deal with the consequences if our own humanity is fully revealed.

Snow & Willard's 1989 study of nurses exposed some of the caring myths. Some 80% of the nurses in their study exhibited 'co-dependence' – a condition of 'lost selfhood ... leading to self-defeating relationships with self and others'. Nurses 'medicate the pain of their disease with alcohol, drugs, food, sex, spending, serial unhappy relationships and more'. In other words, carers may be hooked into the caring relationship like an addiction: we need it, perhaps desperately, to find meaning and purpose in our lives, and we use the caring milieu as a forum to act out all kinds of issues brought with us from our childhood wounds. The caregiver seems just as much in need of caring as the care receiver. The healer is wounded as much as those being helped.

The Nuffield Trust report (Williams et al 1998) suggests that findings such as Snow & Willard's may apply generally to other carers who are finding it difficult to cope. In their efforts to cope, nurses and others fall into the trap of professional 'superhood' – the 'I am in charge of it' attitude which makes it difficult to admit ignorance or show vulnerability. Paradoxically, as Bev Taylor's study (1994) points out, it is not these 'super' men and women, these superdoctors, supernurses and supercarers that patients feel connected with, or from whom they feel they get the best care. It is the 'ordinary' carer, the warm, kind, vulnerable human being that patients feel most at ease with and from whom they feel they get the best care. Furthermore, it has to be remembered that healing relationships are not exclusive to professionals. Just being in the loving presence of another, be it person or animal can make us feel better, and more likely, therefore, to get better. Professionals often hold great store by their apparently unique attributes. Occassionally, a little humility on this theme would not go amiss. A shift of consciousness towards healing does not just happen in the presence of those with lots of health care qualifications. (Plate 2).

Snow & Willard go on to suggest that:

75–90% of nurses bring unresolved issues of co-dependence from their families of origin into their practices in pain-filled overwhelming environments. Is it possible, therefore, that burnout, certain elements of the nursing shortage, professional malaise and addictions to chemicals, food, sex and unhealthy relationships are related largely to nurses hiding their co-dependence issues under the veil of loving and caring for others?

If we replace the word 'nurse' in this statement with the name of any other professional or lay carer, some of the difficulties ring true and are common to all. Behind the veil of caring worn by so many, lies the wounded healer, struggling to cope with his or her own difficulties and limitations, exacerbated by an inhospitable workplace or inadequate resources. These difficult environments may themselves be the products of our failure to connect at a deeper and more meaningful level – to enter into right relationship with our patients and clients, our work colleagues, and ourselves.

Modern health care has seen the retreat of the starched apron and white coat in efforts to be less formal and more accessible to patients. Yet it seems that many of us continue to wear that steely uniform within. It separates us from our patients, and we feel that without that distance, things might fall apart. In his poem 'The Second Coming', W B Yeats wrote:

Turning and turning in the widening gyre
The falcon cannot hear the falconer;
Things fall apart; the centre cannot hold…

Where is our centre that we need to hold on to if we are to be available to others in the world, without suffering ourselves? Where is the centre from which we can move out into the world and build trusting relationships and organisations that help and heal wounds rather than aggravate them? When we as carers suffer burnout and stress, a significant cause may be something that is going on within ourselves, something that feeds the dysfunctional systems and organisations that are constructed all around us. Could it be that without 'a faith in a power greater than ourselves – greater than our parents, our partners, our jobs, our patients – we have difficulty with relationships that operate on other than surface levels' (Snow & Willard 1989)? If work is our centre, but it fails us, for whatever reason, then we have literally lost our faith. The centre no longer holds and we may fall apart – showing all the signs and symptoms of stress and burnout, addiction and co-dependence. Maybe there is another, safer centre that can hold for us. In order to discover that centre, that safe sacred space from which we can be in the world as a healing and caring presence, we need first to explore the relevance of spirituality to the carer.

REFERENCES

Almberg B, Grafstrom M, Winblad B 1997 Caring for the demented elderly person – burden and burnout among caregiving relatives. Journal of Advanced Nursing 25:109–116

Angelou M 1994 Wouldn't take nothing for my journey now. Virago, London

Audit Commission 1998 Finders keepers – the management of staff turnover in NHS trusts. Audit Commission, London

Borrill C F, Wall T D, West G A, Hardy G E et al 1998 Mental health of the workforce in NHS trusts. Institute of Work Psychology, University of Sheffield

Boseley S 1998 Alarm over junior doctors' drug abuse. The Guardian, 4 September, p 2

Campbell A V 1984 Moderated love. SPCK, London

Confederation of British Industry 1991 Promoting mental health at work. CBI, London

Dossey L 1995 Whatever happened to the healers? Alternative Therapies in Health and Medicine 1(5):6–10

Frank A 1991 At the will of the body. Houghton Mifflin, Boston

Griffiths A, Cox T, Stokes A 1995 Work related stress and the law: the current position. Employment Law and Practice 2(4):93–96

Health Education Authority 1996 Organisational stress. HEA, London

Henwood M 1998 Ignored and invisible? Carers' experience of the NHS. Carers National Association, London

Kapur N, Borrill C, Stride C 1998 Psychological morbidity and job satisfaction in hospital consultants and junior house officers: multicentre cross-sectional survey. British Medical Journal 317: 511–512

Mazhindu D 1998 Emotional healing. Nursing Times 94(6):26–31

Princess Royal Trust 1998 Taken for granted? PRT, London

Professions Allied to Medicine 1998 Staff quit NHS. Cited in The Guardian, 8 September, p. 10

Ram Dass, Gorman P 1990 How can I help? Knopf, New York

Salvage J 1985 The politics of nursing. Heinemann, London

Snow C, Willard P 1989 I'm dying to take care of you. Professional Counsellor Books, Redmond

Stapley L F 1996 The personality of the organisation: a psycho-dynamic explanation of culture and change. Free Association Books, London

Taylor B J 1994 Being human – ordinariness in nursing. Churchill Livingstone, Edinburgh

Williams S, Michie S, Pattani S 1998 Improving the health of the NHS workforce. Nuffield Trust, London

World Health Organization 1994 Guidelines for the primary prevention of mental, neurological and psychosocial disorders (5) – Staff Burnout. Ref: WHO/MNH/MND/94.21 WHO Division of Mental Health, Geneva

2

Caring in spirit

> That is at the bottom the only courage that is demanded of us: to
> have courage for the most strange, the most singular and the most
> inexplicable that we may encounter. That mankind has in this sense
> been cowardly has done life endless harm; the experiences that are
> called 'visions', the whole so-called 'spirit world', death, all those
> things that are so closely akin to us, have by daily parrying been so
> crowded out by life that the senses with which we could have
> grasped them are atrophied. To say nothing of God.
>
> *Rainer Maria Rilke*

HUMAN, ALL TOO HUMAN

The humanistic perspective has come to dominate much of western thinking, and is particularly noticeable in the education of professional carers. It can be defined as an outlook or system of thought that is concerned with human rather than divine or supernatural matters. Such a world-view emphasises common human needs and rational ways of solving human problems. People are seen as rational beings whose intellect enables them to act responsibly. The humanist view has its roots deep in western culture – from the ancient Greek and Roman philosophers through to Descartes and subsequent philosophers of the 'Age of Enlightenment' and on to modern humanist therapists, philosophers and psychologists such as Rogers, Maslow, Fromm, Heidegger, Sartre and Marx. Although many of the founders of modern healthcare approaches, and especially of the professions, were devoutly religious people, such as Florence Nightingale, many of today's professional theorists have almost totally rejected this view, preferring the rationalist, humanist approach. In this chapter, we shall examine some of the implications for carers of a philosophical perspective which sees human beings as simply ending at our skin. Humanism's recognition of our personal, but finite existence connecting to others through our interpersonal relationships, perhaps limits the possibilities of what it is to be fully human. The denial of the existence of non-ordinary realities or of transpersonal experience, it will be argued, has led much of healthcare into an inadequate paradigm that fails to meet the demands of holistic care. Furthermore, as we suggested in Chapter 1, the implications spread into the everyday world of the carer, contributing to high levels of stress and burnout. If we, our work or the organisation are the objects of our 'faith', then our faith, and hence our health, can be lost when those 'gods' fail us. The tendency of humanism and secular materialism to sort personhood into physical, social and psychological compartments – spiritual and metaphysical matters tending to be lumped under psychological problems – makes problems for any carer who constantly deals with suffering and death or the existence of an afterlife – issues of primary concern to patients. The impact is not only felt by patients, but also by ourselves as we struggle to bring meaning and purpose to our work. If this life is all there is, how can we cope with the endless suffering that we face each day? If humanism has helped to teach us respect for persons and the notions of human rights and responsibilities, which have helped us to deliver good-quality care, has it also led us to omit whole dimensions of the human experience (of ourselves and our patients) that produce serious difficulties for us when they are not addressed?

THE SPIRIT OF CARING

The bodies were just machines we were taught to mend. Very intricate machines it's true, but machines none the less. All we had to do was apply our complex knowledge, tweak the machine a little here with a drug, there a little with surgery and 'bingo' – it would all sort itself out! In medical school it all seemed so easy in that respect. No extraneous matters to worry about. Then I began to realise that people just didn't seem to fit in with this. Bodies reacted in unpredictable ways despite the certainty of my diagnoses and treatments. I found myself avoiding looking at some people when I knew there was little I could do, they had such faith in me to get it all right and I became more and more aware of just how little I could really do. And then there were the difficult questions – about hope and living and dying and an afterlife. I'd hardly thought about such things myself, let alone had a view to offer someone else. Anyway, such things could easily be tidied away under labels like psychoses, anxiety states, bad after-effects of drugs, endorphins in the brain or whatever. And I used to think, well, if this is all there is, what's the point? Why am I doing this? Will I end up like this some day? There has to be more, there has to be, it can't just be me and them here in this well of suffering. 'Just this' is not enough for me, and it certainly isn't enough for most people who've passed through my hands.

Although much of modern healthcare seems to have lost a sense of the sacred – in its often inhospitable environments and organisations, in the disconnectedness and lack of relationship between colleagues and patients, and the seeming lack of reverence for life and human needs in the face of cost controls – there is still something going on, but we seem to rarely speak of it. Each time we reach out in an act of compassion, with each expression of human caring, with each touch of kindness, the spirit of healthcare is illuminated.

We have built the work of most caring professions on ever more scientific foundations, reinforced by what today is called 'evidence-based practice'. Florence Nightingale is often cited as a noble example of basing work on evidence – from her comments on nursing to recommendations for new sewers. She had mastered the skill of argument based on sound research, but this did not lead her to deny the inspiration for her work, an inspiration which defies scientific explanation – her belief that she was guided by God.

But as Reverend David Stoter (1995) suggests, 'to see spiritual care only as religious care limits its true nature and tends to relegate it to a footnote at the end of the ward report, or something to be handed on to another professional.'

Despite the dominance of the humanistic paradigm in much of modern healthcare literature, education and practice, certain spiritual values and practices seem to have been retained.

> With the work I carry out with my colleagues in my clinical base in our local hospital, I participate in countless acts of compassion every shift. The nurses may not be dropping to their knees in regular bouts of prayer, but they (we) are bringing support, understanding and loving action into every patient encounter, though we may often not be conscious of it. Many would argue that such a service in the day-by-day and night-by-night world of caring work is divinely inspired. The nurses and doctors may not adhere to or acknowledge a particular religious faith, but the service of caring for another human being with compassion is a spiritual act.

Spirituality implies an underpinning belief that people matter, not least ourselves, and in this, it has much in common with the humanistic view. Indeed, some might define humanism as a form of spirituality because it is a belief system that brings meaning and purpose to a particular world-view. Another spiritual perspective tends to add to this view by arguing that acts of caring for the other transcend the here and now. That there may be a deeper purpose and meaning to caring, whether acknowledged or not, which underpins caring actions and intent.

In much of the literature on caring, God and love are a couple of words that are almost absent, and many healthcare professionals seem to have difficulty considering these two themes in their practice. Perhaps driven by the need to appear rational and scientific, or perhaps wary of bringing judgementalism and bigotry into the healthcare setting, we seem collectively to have created a category of taboo words that largely remain outside intellectual debate and practical application in caring.

> We had been caring for this young man for several months. He knew he was dying, and we had all gone through a very traumatic time with him and his family. When J, a new nurse to the unit, started work, there was a discernible shift in staff relationships, but if that had been all, I could have just let it go. She belonged to a particular religious sect, and she seemed unable to have any sort of conversation without expressing her opinion, telling us what her interpretation of the Bible said. Then the complaints started. Two patients were angry, very angry, at her suggestion that their illness was a judgement from God. Another man who died, was laid out by J afterwards, and I found a Bible set across his chest. Mr R was an atheist to the last, and I felt affronted for him. I don't have any problem with religion, I have my own very strong views, but I draw the line at bringing them so bluntly and explicitly into caring for patients unless they want it. She was completely out of line as far as I was concerned, and the atmosphere when we tried to deal with this, first of all face-to face, then going through the managers, was unpleasant to say the least. Eventually J left, but she wrote a

nasty departing letter to us all, saying how we were all godless and doomed to burn in the fires of hell, but that she forgave us. I'm sure she had some personal problems, but it's that sort of thing that gives religion a bad name.

Many authors, such as Alastair Campbell (1984), have described caring as a form of love, albeit with certain conditions attached. Indeed it could be argued that caring requires us to act with unconditional love for another in order to help and heal. Each time we reach out to comfort a crying child, hold the hand of a dying or suffering person or put in that bit of extra effort to make sure a patient gets what she needs, we are performing an act of love. Standing up for the voiceless, the homeless and the disadvantaged, or arguing the case for the services a loved-one needs, or making sure that an injection is given safely and painlessly, or struggling to meet the needs of drunken or violent patients in an accident and emergency department when we might be scared or trying to suppress our rejection of them – all these take love.

However, without that loving connection to another human being – which some argue (Mother Meera 1991, Rodegast & Stanton 1987) is difficult if not impossible to achieve without an acceptance of the divine within each of us – it is too easy to disconnect, to see the other person as an 'it'. Martin Buber (1937) considers two distinct human approaches to others: 'I–It' and 'I–Thou'. When we consider somebody as an 'it', separation from us is implied, allowing us to adopt all manner of malicious behaviour, as the evidence of abuse of vulnerable people shows through the ages. If we approach the world from a perspective that 'this is all there is', it can provoke us always to give of our best in what little time we have available to us, but conversely, it may bring out the worst: if this is all there is, why not exploit everyone, the planet included, and make my own life as comfortable as I can while it lasts? This view is encapsulated in a Peggy Lee song from the 1960s:

> If that's all there is, my friends,
> then let's keep dancing.
> Let's break out the booze and have a ball
> If that's all there is.
>
> *(Peggy Lee, Columbia Records, 1969)*

A spiritual perspective finds deeper meanings. When we accept the essential equal value and divinity of the other, we relate to them as 'thou' (Buber 1937), we do to them as we do to ourselves, for we are all connected, all part of each other. Such compassionate behaviour transcends person and situation, but is not necessarily easily achieved. It is relatively easy to see the love of God if we sit and contemplate the images of our particular faith but it is much more difficult to see that same divine connection in a mass murderer or child abuser. It's easy to love a pleasant patient but much more difficult if she is nasty to us or has committed a wicked act.

People often ask me: how can you work with these people? They have murdered, committed terrible crimes, are subject to widespread public hatred. They can behave abominably to you, sometimes violent, aggressive, ungrateful, unpredictable. I don't have an easy answer to that. I know that they all have one thing in common, usually a very nasty upbringing, but even that sounds like an excuse. I just know that, while what they have done may be terrible, they are human beings with their own needs, their own pain and struggles. They are deserving of my help, my compassion, because they are here, because there but for the grace of God go I, because, well I don't know what else, just because. They are just suffering human beings like others, and because I am human too, how or why should I turn my back on them? Suffering is suffering wherever you find it, it doesn't matter to me how bad or good the people seem to be. More than that, if I were to reject them then I'm not sure that I could live with myself. It would be as if I had somehow also turned my back on me. I don't like or approve of much of what they have done, but they are still human beings, just like me.

What we seem to struggle with is understanding the nature of that love, where it comes from, and how it affects us and our patients. We tend to view love through the narrow lens of soap opera emotions such as lust, or attachment to people or things, and so we could be forgiven for being confused or reticent when impersonal love is used in a caring context, what is often called 'agape' – a non-sexual compassionate caring for another, regardless of who they are or what they have done, and which recognises the fundamental value and perhaps divinity of each of us. When we do that, when we make that connection, caring for others, no matter who we perceive them to be or what they have done, can be accomplished with equity and equanimity. When we see the divine not only in ourselves but others, we are no longer separate. In caring for the other, one cares also for oneself. It is this transcendent quality of non-judgemental caring, whether explicit or not, that has underpinned caring ideals for centuries. Such caring love for another is an act of spirituality, a sacred thing in itself.

However, it must be remembered that there are risks for us when we give love. As Chapter 1 has illustrated, each act of compassion and caring can leave us drained and burned out when we rely upon the little islands of ourselves for its source, a tendency reinforced by the humanistic perspective of 'there is only me'. Perhaps the answer is not so much to exhaust ourselves *doing* compassion, giving constantly of our own resources, but rather to *become* and *be* compassion – to relax into being available and allow the love to simply do its healing work (Ram Dass & Bush 1992). To be able to do this, we need to accept that there is a greater realm of being than the brief flash of our existence in this world, that there is something greater within us and beyond us that brings meaning, understanding and compassion to our often nightmarish work, something which enables us to 'keep our hearts open in hell' (Ram Dass & Gorman 1990). A purely humanistic perspective may limit us here, for if we acknowledge the existence of nothing but our physical reality, we have only the strength of that reality to draw on.

SPIRITUALITY

In western cultures especially, we worship at the altar of the rationalist paradigm, largely attributed to the thinking of Descartes and his followers, where everything can be reduced to logic, quantity and observable evidence, and mind and body are separate and soul denied. However, it is worth noting that many great rationalists and scientists close to that age (such as Descartes and, later, Newton) were devoutly religious people. Yet what was subsequently built on their thinking has often turned away from any suggestion of the possibility of a transpersonal human dimension. Many healthcare systems throughout the world have witnessed the impact of the entirely rationalist-positivist view – questioning approaches based on tradition or the service ethic as more and more demands are made for cost control and hard, evidence-based practice from healthcare workers. Jones (1996) remarks that:

For the last two hundred years, Western culture has been an experiment to test the hypothesis that human beings can be totally fulfilled in an atmosphere of secular rationalism, technological efficiency, and material abundance alone. Evidence for the falsity of the claim that we can live without meaning daily pours into the psychotherapists' offices. We see the anomie and emptiness symptomatic of the ethos with its disconnection from anything smacking of value, purpose, or the experience of the sacred.

For Snow & Willard (1989), whose fascinating study we cited in Chapter 1, spirituality transcends the limitations of human mind and body, it 'assures us that we are not alone', that 'we do not have to be in control of others' – thereby allowing us to 'trust, to be honest and therefore vulnerable, and to live in acceptance of ourselves and others' and to share a 'faith in a power greater than ourselves'. For some people spirituality simply suggests a connection with the deeper meaning and purpose of life, and does not necessarily mean acceptance of the divine. For others, coming home to a relationship with God, in whatever way the divine is perceived, is what a spiritual journey is all about.

An exclusively humanistic and scientific perspective, though, leaves little room for other than people: only we can be in control. The reduced world of 'just me and nothing else' feeds the need to be in control of everything, from the climate to the production of children. Jones (1996) goes on to note that fear of losing control seems to be one of the major symptoms of our age: 'Many an ulcer, hypertensive, or anxiety attack begins when contemporary men and women sense their lives slipping out of control', and this in turn lies at the root of many illnesses and a 'close-mindedness about spiritual experience'.

The WHO long ago defined health as a state of complete physical and mental wellbeing rather than merely the absence of disease (WHO 1948). If, as will be argued, spirituality and our deep hunger for connection and for the sacred are fundamental to our sense of wellbeing, then the WHO definition seems to have omitted a crucial element of what it is to be healthy. The WHO seem to have recognised this omission in recent guidance, redefining health as 'a dynamic state of complete physical, mental, spiritual and social wellbeing' and not merely the absence of disease (WHO 1998). Perhaps we are also sick, dis-eased, when we are not in a state of complete wellbeing spiritually.

The need to find purpose and meaning in life is not just a feature of those who are sick or close to death. It is a universal trait necessary for the maintenance of life and part of a well-developed personality. Thus it seems possible to argue, that if we have not deepened our understanding of our place in the scheme of things and our spiritual roots, we may be seen as more prone to being dis-eased or unhealthy. Likewise, carers who have no clear understanding of their own spirituality is arguably less able to care for others in whom there is a need for spiritual support. Time and again throughout the literature on spirituality, we encounter a repeating theme: that spirituality is a kind of rock-hard centre within ourselves, a place of solidity and certainty in an uncertain world full of complexity and uncertainty. It provides both map and compass, as well as the ship to guide us through life. Those embedded in such a world-view seem better able to care for others, to be more available without judgementalism or the need to control, and better able to take care of themselves and their own health (Benson 1996).

If spirituality is part of our health, what is it that makes it so different? Jones (1996) sees spirituality as 'tuning the spirit within us to its source' and Kelting (1995) believes that this desire to be attuned lives in all of us and comments that we 'hunger for a sense of purpose, destiny and value, grounded not only in ourselves, but in the wider nature of things. We also seek comfort and love, not just for and from one another, but for and from the greater realm of being'. O'Brien (1982) defines spirituality as that which inspires in one the desire to transcend the realm of the material'. Dr Lauren Artress, Canon of Grace Cathedral in San Francisco, who has done much to restore the use of labyrinths as a spiritual tool (see Ch. 4) sees spirituality as the 'inward activity of growth and maturation that happens in each of us', whereas religion is the outward form, the 'container', specifically the liturgy and all the acts of worship that teach, praise, and give thanks to God' (Artress 1995). Religion is

another vehicle for the expression of spirituality ... channelled through such avenues as prayers, rituals, religious communities and worship. The institution codifies and provides pathways for the expression of beliefs and values held by the person. It provides meaning in the day to day chores of life, and sustains the person through personal hardships such as illness, pain and personal disaster. It provides an avenue for celebration when personal hardships are overcome (Labun 1988).

Religion and spirituality are thus intertwined and, for many, the difference is meaningless, religion having provided a focus for spiritual expression and creating the context for spirituality to emerge. However, it is important to remember that, while everyone may be spiritual (needing and pursuing a deeper understanding of themselves, their place in the cosmos and, perhaps, their relationships with the divine) not everyone is religious (following their spirituality through a specific system of beliefs and practices). Moreover, the union is not always a happy one. Most religions have, historically, tried at some point to suppress any individual expression of spirituality that challenges accepted dogma. Some commentators approaching from a humanistic perspective (e.g. Storr 1996) have dismissed the religious and spiritual pursuit as a psychiatric phenomenon, a search for security and a father or authority figure in a difficult world. In the 19th century, Nietzsche, having famously declared that 'God is dead', saw the loss of belief as a great opportunity to voyage on the 'open sea' of humanity without the restraint of religious dogma. Humanism, the belief in the essential value and power of every human being, was in part a reaction to religious orthodoxy and fundamentalism. However, as human values tend to shift with time and circumstance, there may be risks when moral relativism emerges. This can be witnessed in the debates which rage over such issues as euthanasia, abortion and genetic screening.

Recent thinking and research into physics, spirituality and psychology are pointing towards a new understanding of consciousness and energy, demonstrating an awesome unity and pattern in the universe which is far from impersonal or neutral. Much of this new thinking has failed so far to get through to our medical and nursing schools and teachers, many of whom remain hooked on reductionist biological, psychological or sociological models of human beings. Long ago, Isaac Newton, regarded as one of the founders of the scientific age, yet also a deeply religious man, acknowledged that the more he understood the nature of things, the more he was convinced of a greater power and purpose that lay behind it. Similar viewpoints can be found in the writings of many other great scientists, from Einstein to Hawking. Perhaps then we do not have to think in terms of science *or* spirituality, but of science *and* spirituality. The new humanism of the post-modern era is being pushed into embracing transpersonal phenomena, and a new model may be emerging. Or rather, we may be rediscovering an ancient model, to which modern science is lending new credibility in a secular world. The notion of a universe where everything is interconnected and united by the same force of energy as described by modern physics would not be out of place in ancient spiritual texts or the view of any mystic (Plate 3).

This point is illustrated in the writings of Skolimowski (1992), a philosopher and ecologist from whose work the notion of ecopraxis has emerged. He is particularly scathing about modern philosophy, which he sees as having little to say about the wider world, the cosmos and our connection to it as human beings. For the carer, this means living and working in the world in ways that are 'sensitive to environments, to vibrational energy fields' and seeing oneself 'as compassionate in relation to everything else'. This 'ecological person's' spirituality embraces sensitivities such as 'logic, intuition, morality, aesthetics and a sense of the sacred'. Being 'cocreators, we are capable of moving to a higher order in their (our) lives, guided by moral codes …. Ecophilosophy …

depicts a view that is life-orientated, and about the interconnectedness of all things, compassionately united with the flow of life in the universe'. Such a view of our place in the cosmos is echoed in thinking on spirituality both ancient and modern. From the Upanishads to Einstein, the notion of the interconnectedness of all things in the universe, ourselves included, provides the ethical thrust for our compassionate concern for ourselves, others and the world. When we recognise our place in the awesome history of evolution and the cosmos, when we see ourselves as a strand in the web that connects us all, it is difficult not to be reverential towards all of creation.

To the Native Americans, such a spiritual path is nothing new. The Navajo nation see the spiritual path as 'walking the beauty way' – living in the grace of the wonder of the universe, and having reverence for all of creation. A 'coming home' to our own spirituality, seeing ourselves as part of the whole (see also Ch. 5), enables us to let go of so many of the 'ties that bind'. It helps us facilitate the health of others, and in so doing to be healthy ourselves. The word 'health' has its roots in the Teutonic 'hal' (in Old English 'hælan') meaning whole, hale or holy. Our health and that of others are intimately connected to our desire to be whole. It is not possible to be whole without the appreciation of our unique part in the Whole.

> My own experience is still unfolding, often blissful, sometimes painful. I know too that it is shared by many other nurses the more I find myself willing to open up and discuss it more freely. There seems to be a considerable degree of collective denial among my nursing and medical colleagues, that is only shed in private conversation or hushed tones. A very experienced and well-known nurse recently confided in me at a major conference. I had been relating some of my own experiences and beliefs, and the response was 'yes, that's happened to me too, but I don't talk about it. I think you shouldn't either, they'll just think you're mad.' I suspect this spiritual awakening and awareness is happening to far more people than is generally acknowledged. It falls outside conventional religious arenas and I suspect that large numbers of people feel that it's something odd that might only be happening to them. We can talk about sex and death now in polite society. Perhaps it's time for us to bring God out of the closet.

THE SPIRITUAL JOURNEY

The spiritual journey is not without risk, as will be discussed in more detail in Chapter 5. No two people seem to experience exactly the same path, and religions have tended to suppress personal spiritual exploration, partly because of the personal risks involved, but also in efforts to retain control and impose orthodoxy. For many religions, this produces a dilemma, precisely because this suppression of the individual relationship with the divine leads many people to satisfy their spiritual hunger in places other than churches, temples or mosques. Such people may fall under the spell of cults and gurus (Storr 1996) or lose direction in the welter of options available in the modern-day 'spiritual supermarket'. Spiritual experiences can be profound and life-transforming, but they can be interpreted by others as madness (witness Joan of Arc, for example), especially when they lead to behaviour that prevents us from being socially grounded and able to function in the everyday world. There seems to be a great and growing hunger for a spiritual connection in our culture, a hunger that the orthodox religions often seem unable to satisfy. The pain of this hunger for the sacred in ourselves is a dulled by many with drink or drugs, as we suggested in Chapter 1. As the effects wear off, we return to face the very thing that we tried to escape, or we lose the connection we thought we found under their influence. Other people feel the need to withdraw from the world for a while, but this can shatter relationships or lead to isolation. In a speech in Manchester in 1996, the Dalai Lama reminded the audience that a personal spiritual quest may or may not require a retreat *from* the physical world for a time. However, it is quite a different quest when our intention is to activate love and compassion for the purpose of relieving suffering *in* the world.

It is suggested in many opinion polls that Europe in general, and the UK in particular, is still predominantly Christian, and the majority of people when asked, described themselves, at least loosely, as Christian. However, the exodus from our churches continues unabated, and vicars and priests regularly complain that they only see their parishioners at births, marriages and funerals. Storr (1996) notes how less than 2.5% of the population regularly attend church on Sunday, and cites the Bishop of Oxford's comment that 'We in western Europe are now in a post-Christian society'. Other religions appear to be capitalising to some degree on this exodus, yet they too may have their problems in maintaining membership and orthodoxy. Meanwhile a whole tranche of mix-and-match cults and personal approaches often loosely described as 'New Age' is fuelling this decline. Perhaps part of the problem, as in healthcare, is the loss of the spiritual tradition. Dogma, observance of form and ritual, obsession with systems, structures and outcomes and the limited perspective of humanism, sterilises the spiritual context. To paraphrase T S Eliot's *Four Quartets*, we 'have the experience, but miss the meaning'. If Christianity is to survive (and the same may apply to other religions) perhaps there is a need to return to a deeper exploration of its mystical and spiritual roots, a revival of the personal experience of a spiritual journey. Perhaps that experience of the personal and spiritual, bringing meaning and understanding to the world of work, is what is missing from healthcare as well.

However, it is questionable if this can be rectified through a return, as some have suggested (e.g. Bradshaw 1994), to what is perceived as a golden age of certainty of the Christian covenant in healthcare. In times of uncertainty, there is a tendency to hark back to old certainties which runs the risk of lapsing into fundamentalism and rigid dogma, even if it were possible to go back. (Florence Nightingale herself (quoted in Poovey 1991) said that 'the law of God it seems, is against repetition'). Such an approach has its roots in fear, not love of the divine. Religion clearly still has a place and significance for many patients and carers, the rituals and forms helping immensely through times of suffering. But is there more to it than this? What about all of those for whom religion, where it has become alienated from spirituality, ceases to have meaning, usefulness or purpose?

THE RATIONAL MODEL IN HEALTHCARE

The objectification of health has led us to a point of great concern for healthcare and the carer. Some aspects of care, which do not lend themselves easily to measurement or evaluation, can find themselves excluded. This applies particularly to the 'softer' services such as some of the complementary therapies, counselling and chaplaincy.

> I'd gone through the whole range of orthodox treatments for my breast cancer, and after several years, I was basically told that nothing more could be done. 'You can go home and die now' was the unspoken message. I was determined not to let it go at that. There had to be more, alternatives that I had not tried, treatments that the established doctors didn't know about. The Gerson diet I am using now is healthy, full of organic produce and fresh vegetables and fruit, but it's very expensive. I've had a running battle with the medical establishment to seek funding and support for something that has certainly helped me feel better, which may cure me, and I feel has certainly kept me alive longer after they had washed their hands of me. But it just doesn't fit with their way of thinking … they want research, hard evidence. As with so many of these things, there's not much there. But I'm here, so what more evidence do they need?

The Cartesian, rational, scientific, humanistic, essentially masculine world-view has struck healthcare worldwide this past decade as never before. As healthcare systems struggle to contain costs – and sometimes fall apart – there is an ever greater struggle to identify certainty amid a sense of threat, challenge and insecurity. Worshipping at the altar of cost-effectiveness, those who control the systems increasingly sideline many aspects of caring which cannot be proved to be 'evidence-based'. The knock-on effects are serious. There is a tendency, for example, to justify 'rationing' of healthcare (euphemistically referred to as 'prioritising', 'downsizing', 're-engineering') and to apportion it accordingly to the deserving and the undeserving (the latter group usually consisting of elderly people, the chronically ill, the disabled and so on). Furthermore, the focus tends to be exclusively on actions which are observable and measurable – 'instrumental skills' (Benner 1984), even though much of caring is 'invisible' (Lawler 1991) and difficult, if not impossible, to measure. The compassion of carer for patient has meaning and significance for both, but how can this be quantified any more than counting the pleasure we get from hearing a symphony, the sense of wellbeing from being among loved ones, or the inspiration that may come from a great work of art or poetry? If it cannot be measured, the risk is that it will not be paid for in a system that recognises only tasks, measurable actions and outcomes.

Within the caring professions themselves, this objectification is producing a class of people who subscribe to the view that the rationalist–scientific model is all that matters. In some realms of healthcare research and academia, for example, in order to appear rational and scientific, to gain social acceptance within this world-view, the elite have distanced themselves from the reality of caring practice. Sogyal Rinpoche (1992) summarises this view:

Our contemporary education indoctrinates us in the glorification of doubt, has created in fact what could almost be called a religion or theology of doubt, in which to be seen to be intelligent we have to be seen to doubt everything, to always point to what's wrong and rarely to ask what's right or good, cynically to denigrate all inherited ideals and philosophies, or any theory that is done in simple goodwill or an innocent heart.

When old values and certainties are challenged, we may look into the narcissistic mirror offered by others to bring certainty into an uncertain world. Science, technology, reason – these appear to offer such certainties, a centre that holds. However, this model is only half adequate for caring. So much else in caring relies upon meaning, intuition, feelings, upon how we *are* with patients, not what we *do* to them. Joseph Campbell (1988) reminds us: 'Technology is not going to save us. Our computers, our tools, our machines are not enough. We have to rely on our intuition, our true being'.

This true being can only be discovered in the spiritual search, and to do this we must look internally as well as externally for our reference points for caring. As was suggested in Chapter 1, when things go wrong, we often look for short-term solutions: change the system, introduce new procedures, get rid of the difficult manager. Perhaps the focus on external change (form), giving the impression that we are improving things, is a sign not so much of our success but of our insecurity, our inability to face what is really going on inside and what we really need to deal with. The external activities may be not so much evidence of our success in improving care, but of denial. We look to the outer because the inner is too difficult and painful to bear. However, without a sound basis of inner-centredness and certainty, the outer lacks substance, feels uncentred and is dehumanised. It contains the head but not the heart of caring, and fails as a result. The outer manifestations of caring may be taking place, but something seems to be missing. It may be difficult to pin down and identify, and it may be that we know it by its absence rather than its presence. Patients especially are sensitive to it, though it may be difficult for them to articulate or make explicit. People can feel cared for, but not cared about. Carers go through the motions of caring, giving the injections, the sound advice, the hot baths, but some other dimension – conveying that the person is valued, loved even – is left out. Enough patients in the orthodox healthcare system seem to sense this, if the evidence from the escalating level of complaints and the increasing use of complementary and alternative therapies is anything to go by. And enough carers sometimes sense this too. Feeling unable to give care the way they 'know' it should be done, they form part of the mass exodus from the orthodox professions into complementary therapies or other work. In contexts bereft of a spiritual core, some struggle to integrate holistic practices into their way of working, while others move on in the hope of finding or creating that safe sacred space in which their ideals can be fulfilled. However, the picture is not all bleak – there are signs of change, significant change, which we will discuss later.

Meanwhile, to suggest that there is a spiritual malaise among healthcare workers or informal carers is seen as contentious. It is not politically correct, in the UK, for example, to suggest that carers are not coping. To do so would imply that our systems are not as good as they might be, that resources to help the home carer need improving, that time, money and effort might need to be spent. Furthermore, the 'internal' is seen as too private – leave well alone, do not disturb the defence mechanisms. This ostrich-like syndrome (a form of denial) assumes that there is no problem and that the carers can cope, without explaining the high suicide, co-dependency and attrition rates explored in Chapter 1.

While not denying the need for continued external change, it may be that there are other areas of change that we now must face. These changes may be internal as well as external, and may feel risky. This is not least, as we shall see in subsequent chapters, because the subject can be interpreted as a spiritual sickness in the individual. Therefore it is the individual's problem, and society, governments and organisations can safely wash their hands of it. However, some of the strategies for change are relatively straightforward. Providing support for staff at a wider organisational level, among the team at local/unit level and through personal strategies such as meditation, exercise, counselling and time out, are examples of simple things that can be done. We will be exploring these strategies in Chapter 3.

More enlightened organisations are already moving in this direction, not least because investing in carers in this way is seen as cost-effective. It is interesting to note that arguments about cost-effectiveness can be the very cause of a shift to a greater consideration of spirituality and supportive strategies for carers. Many of the arguments for altering staffing levels, working practices and so on have relied upon convincing evidence of cost-effectiveness and controls. Increasing evidence from the same rationalist – positivist approach to healthcare is now emerging which justifies expenditure on what has often previously been dismissed as the emotive, qualitative or irrelevant aspects of caring. The Scientific approach is now being used to look at the 'softer' side of healthcare and is helping to shift the debate towards cost-effective arguments in this field as well. The tools, once seen by many as undermining the qualitative aspects of caring, are now causing us to appreciate them. Thus, a second area in need of attention is the current focus on the rational–scientific, which needs to be balanced by the intuitive–caring aspect. This is not a question of either/or, but of both. When we rely solely on factual, linear, research-guided models of care, we may fail to integrate intuitive principles which move us towards healing. These principles are 'feelings, ways of knowing answers to problems that either are not provable or defy scientific law. When applied to Western healing practices, alternative healing methods – certain forms of touch, energy balancing, psychic skills – often make no sense. Yet they work' (Snow & Willard 1989). And so a rebalancing of healing skills, of masculine and feminine perspectives, is seen as essential to the restoration of healing in healthcare generally.

RIGHT RELATIONSHIP

Spirituality is, as we have shown, fundamental to right relationship with ourselves, others and beyond. Without it, we may live in a world bereft of heart and meaning. Schumacher (1977) notes:

A person, for instance, entirely fixed in the philosophy of materialistic scientism, denying the reality of the 'invisibles' and confining his attention solely to what can be counted, measured and weighed, lives in a very poor world, so poor that he will experience it as a meaningless wasteland unfit for human habitation. Equally, if he sees it as nothing but an accidental collocation of atoms he will needs agree with Bertrand Russell that the only rational attitude is one of 'unyielding despair'.

In other words, part of the malaise in caring relationships may be an inner one, a loss of acceptance of the Divine, to look beyond ourselves or society for our moral guidance or codes of practice.

Unfortunately, in the face of unyielding despair, when fears stalk us – fears about our work, about society, ourselves – we tend to return to old certainties or rigid rules. This echoes our discussion of spirituality and religion: in the search for certainty, religion often risks lapsing into dogma and fundamentalism. (We will look at some aspects of this in relation to the shadow side of the sacred in Ch. 5.) Such narrow thinking, however, denies the pluralistic nature of the modern world. A new paradigm, a new blueprint of how we see the world, which embraces the spiritual, seems to be emerging. Carey (1991), for example, argues: 'To choose religious or ideological dogmatism in the name of freedom is as foolish as for a jailed man to exercise his right to remain in prison'. There is no going back, and adherence to any dogma, religious or humanistic, may only limit rather than liberate us.

An enormous amount of attention is paid to changing systems, structures and organisations. This may be only half the story. Perhaps we need to focus on getting the relationships right first. When relationships are right, everything else falls into place and the systems work. Right relationships – with each other, ourselves, our organisations and perhaps with our God – will re-energise and revitalise who we are and what we do and give meaning and value to what we bring to our work. Thomas (1983), for example, believes that: 'We do not know enough about ourselves. We are ignorant about how we work, about where we fit in and most of all about the enormous, imponderable system of life in which we are embedded as working parts'.

Meanwhile, Carey (1991) goes on to remind us that, 'You cannot travel into yourself without exploring the infinite reaches of eternal consciousness. You cannot know yourself in reality without knowing God'.

Right relationships begin with ourselves. This exploration will inevitably transcend the very limited scientific view of what we are as human beings, and cause us to re-examine and incorporate spiritual values into our caring work. When this occurs, the healing potential expands. The hospital, for example, could be revived as a place of retreat, nurture, succour and healing, and reoriented away from the modernist revolving-door, clinical sickness machine it has become. New relationships can come into existence which recognise the value of being with people as much as doing to them. Carers can let go of the intense effort required to give compassion, and relax into *being* compassionate, *being* healing, in short, *becoming* the sacred space in which healing occurs. As we suggested in the Introduction, sacred space is illuminated in right relationships. Mark Young (quoted in Forder & Forder 1995), an osteopath and Sufi, has this to say: 'There can be a moment in healing when there is perfect balance and all distinction ... between healer and wounded disappears. It is at this point that something else can enter and both are transported to a place of mystery. Part of us yearns to return to this place, because it is here that we are made whole'. (Plate 4)

When we enter into right relationship, not only with the world and each other, but with ourselves and perhaps our God, then we find that centre where we not only give healing, we become healing. In Chapters 3 and 4, we look at some ways in which we might bring this about.

REFERENCES

Artress L 1995 Walking a sacred path – rediscovering the labyrinth as a sacred tool. Riverhead, New York
Benner P 1984 Novice to expert. Addison Wesley, New York
Benson H 1996 Timeless healing. Simon & Schuster, London
Bradshaw A 1994 Lighting the lamp. Scutari, Harrow
Buber M 1937 I and Thou. T & T Clark, Edinburgh
Campbell A V 1984 Moderated love. SPCK, London
Campbell J 1988 The power of myth. Doubleday, New York
Carey K 1991 The third millennium. Harper, San Francisco
Forder J, Forder E 1995 The light within. Usha Publications, Cumbria
Jones J 1996 In the middle of this road we call our life. Harper Collins, London
Kelting T 1995 The nature of nature. Parabola 20(1): 24–30
Labun E 1988 Spiritual care – an element of nursing practice. Journal of Advanced Nursing 13: 314–320
Lawler J 1991 Behind the screens. Churchill Livingstone, Edinburgh
Mother Meera 1991 Answers. Rider, London
Nightingale F In: Poovey M (ed) 1991 Cassandra-suggestions for thought. Pickering, London
O'Brien M E 1982 The need for spiritual integrity. In: Yura H, Walsh M B (eds) Human needs and the nursing process. Appleton-Century-Crofts, New York
Ram Dass, Bush M 1992 Compassion in action. Bell, New York
Ram Dass & Gorman P 1990 How can I help? Rider, London
Rodegast P, Stanton J 1987 Emmanuel's book. Bantam, New York

Schumacher E F 1977 A guide for the perplexed. Abacus, London
Skolimowski H 1992 Living philosophy: ecophilosphy as a tree of life. Arkana, London
Snow C, Willard P 1989 I'm dying to take care of you. Professional Counsellor Books, Redmond
Sogyal Rinpoche 1992 The Tibetan book of living and dying. Rider, London
Storr A 1996 Feet of clay – a study of gurus. Harper Collins, London
Stoter D 1995 Spiritual aspects of healthcare. Mosby, London
Thomas L 1983 The medusa and the snail. Bantam, New York
World Health Organisation 1948 Constitution of the WHO. WHO, Geneva
World Health Organisation 1998 Definition of Health. WHO, Geneva

3

Sacred space at work

The Myth of Sisyphus
Sisyphus was condemned for his sin. In the underworld, his task
was to roll a huge boulder up a hill. He would painstakingly roll
the boulder slowly up and up almost to the summit, then the rock
would roll out of his grasp and crash right to the bottom. If
Sisyphus could stop and decide never to roll the stone again, he
would have peace.

From Anam Cara by John O'Donohue

In this chapter, we pick up on the three themes touched upon in Chapter 2:
the organisation, the way teams work, and the part played by ourselves.
James Jones (1996) remarks that 'Spirituality is both a theory and a practice.
The words experiment and experience have the same root. Spirituality says,
do certain things and you will experience your connection with the sacred'.
What are the 'certain things' that can be done in these three arenas to restore
the sacred to caring relationships?

RIGHT RELATIONSHIP IN ORGANISATIONS

The use of terms such as 'sacred' or 'spirituality' in the workplace can seem
hopelessly unrealistic. Healthcare is so often dominated by issues of cost and
control and, as we have suggested, the organisations and the caring
relationships themselves may often be sick. Patch Adams (1993), a highly
charismatic doctor who took a very alternative approach to healthcare and
whose life story has been made into a major Hollywood film, remarks that
'the concept of service has become misplaced in the madness of operating
medicine like a business'. Are the ethics of business compatible with the
service ethic? Is making money compatible with caring? Is caring for staff
secondary to getting patients (as cheaply as possible) through the system?

Deepak Chopra (1996) is one eminent doctor who believes that the two do
not have to be incompatible. Running healthcare, if not to make profit, then
at least to cover costs as is the case with most state-funded or cooperative
systems, can be done in a business-like way without necessarily running it
like a business. The worst excesses of the capitalist system, such as maximising
output at the expense of the quality of patient care, exploiting staff or making
all decisions on the grounds of profitability, can be avoided if a new approach
is taken. Chopra notes that many large corporations are now adopting
spiritual principles in order to attain success 'because when you focus on

values, the economic side of life takes care of itself'. In other words, taking care of the staff in an organisation, developing positive working relationships and practices that have heart and meaning for the staff, can be seen as an investment, just like putting more money into the business. Christine Payne (cited in Wright 1993), a former senior nurse in the UK's National Health Service (NHS), observes that getting the relationships right in organisations brings about 'cost benefits' because the whole system works more efficiently: 'money, time and frustration are wasted on dealing with complaints, complications, sickness, absenteeism and so on'. The system works more efficiently with good relationships, saving time and money on 'doing repairs'.

A recent study for the Gallup Organisation reported by Dennis Hatfield (1999), found that companies with high levels of what Daniel Goleman (1995) called 'emotional intelligence' were more likely to be efficient, effective and profitable. Emotional intelligence – the ability of teams or groups to collaborate effectively and harmoniously – emerges as a key determinant of the success of an organisation. 'When two groups are equal in all other factors, (e.g. talent and skill)', remarks Hatfield, 'the group with higher emotional/group intelligence will be more productive and successful'. Once again, we see the nature of relationships in an organisation as the key to its effectiveness:

Employee satisfaction, boosted by such things as good quality relationships with managers and co-workers and respect for their importance, future and connectedness is a direct route to customer satisfaction as well as productivity, profit, reduced turnover and other critical outcomes (Hatfield 1999).

Thus harmonious relationships in the workplace, often seen as a luxurious extra when the 'more important' matters have been dealt with (ensuring the right work patterns and systems are in place) emerges as central and pivotal to an organisation's success.

One of the instruments used by Gallup posed 12 questions to employees. Positive employee perceptions associated with those statements converged strongly with organisational productivity, reduced turnover, profit and customer satisfaction:

1. I know what is expected of me.
2. I have sufficient materials and equipment.
3. I have the opportunity to do what I do best.
4. I have received praise in the last 7 days.
5. My supervisor cares about me.
6. My professional development is encouraged.
7. My opinions seem to count.
8. I understand the mission/purpose of the company.
9. My work associates are committed to quality.
10. My best friend is at work.
11. I have the opportunity to learn and grow.
12. My supervisor has talked with me about my progress.

'Creating a great place to work', Hatfield suggests, involves 'right relationships' where managers 'manage with heart' and nurture 'clear and involving expectations, recognition and a sense of learning and growth'. An absence of right relationships can be likened to the difference between turbulence and laminar flow. Organisations with smooth-running relationships can devote more energy and attention to the quality and effectiveness of the work in hand. Turbulent relationships waste energy and attention, and reduce quality and effectiveness.

Emotional intelligence rooted in right relationships is not fixed like IQ: it can be developed through team building and employee support strategies. Interestingly, Goleman (1995) also believes that spiritual practices can help people towards emotional intelligence, especially with aspects of self-awareness and empathy. In an interview with Michael Toms (1999), Goleman insists that empathy is 'the basis of caring and compassion, which relates to spiritual practice. Spiritual practices may help people develop emotional intelligence within'.

Thus, as we shall discuss further in Chapter 4, there seems to be a place for fostering spiritual practices of individuals. We can see this as one further means of enhancing relationships and, hence, in the case of healthcare workers, for example, better quality and effectiveness at work.

This message has yet to percolate through all healthcare organisations, and many continue to foster cultures of control rather than cooperation, fear rather than love, punishment rather than reward. In such climates, we develop an 'I-It' (Buber 1937) relationship with the workplace, where the workplace is a place where we turn up and go through the motions because we have to, because we need the money, because there is no alternative, or whatever. We feel no investment in it, and more often than not, dislike being there. We find it difficult to give of our best, and are more inclined not to turn up for work or be off sick. In fact, the workplace may actually contribute to us feeling ill in the first place. The 'I-It' view of the world means that we relate to something else – be it a person or a thing – as an object 'out there'. The relationship is one of distance, disconnection and remoteness. Conversely, an 'I-Thou' relationship is held by connection, meaning, purpose, love and understanding in whatever or whoever we relate to. We feel connected to it, wish to see the relationship flourish, draw strength and positive feelings from it ourselves – it has heart and meaning to it. In the case of the workplace, it feels welcoming to both our heart and our soul.

I'd been working on Victoria Ward for 7 years. I felt stuck there, going nowhere. We were just doing the same old routines. It was very regimented. Lots of rules. The patients had to fit in with our system and not the other way round. It was one of those old 'geriatric' wards. Stuck away in an old building at the back of the hospital. The care was unimaginative and very routinised. The sister was OK to work for, you knew where you stood with her, but her rule was law, you just did as you were told and heaven help you if you stepped out of line. Come to think of it, the whole hospital was run like that. What was happening on Victoria was just a miniature version of what the rest of the place was like. Do as you're told. Just come in, bath 'em, wash 'em, feed 'em and go home again. Everything was so controlled, you had to ask permission to sneeze – suggest a change and it was as if you'd sworn in church. Everything had to be the way it was because there was always some problem lurking in the shadows if you were to change it. Yet the place was unhappy. Lots of patient complaints, staff didn't stay long, there always seemed to be somebody off sick, all that sort of thing. But, well, what could you do? To be honest, I didn't know much different. After a while you stop questioning, learn to keep your head down and just get on with it. When S came in and took charge of the place it was like a whirlwind hit. There seemed to be 10 new ideas a day. We started to organise care into different teams, each of us responsible for a different group of patients. We began to bring in new ideas, that I'd read about but always thought they were for other places, not run-of-the-mill units like ours: primary nursing, complementary therapies, pet therapy, patient access to health records, open visiting and meal times, staff out of uniform, new specialist roles, a patients' committee to help run the ward – the list seemed endless. Somehow we all felt liberated, like lots of energy that had been kept bottled up was suddenly let loose. Work became exciting and interesting again. We all began to give far more than we took. We seemed to relate to patients and each other as real people. I'm not sure what it could be put down to, a new leader was certainly a catalyst, but it was certainly more than that. Once he arrived, everything else just seemed to take off, like it had all been waiting in a queue for years and now it had a chance to move forward. We all seemed to be so much more involved. The place became a joy to work in. I began to look forward to going to work again. I just loved being there. Loved being a nurse once more.

Ken Carey (1991) reminds us that 'all human organisations rooted in fear will be faced with increasing structural difficulties until they either change, restructure or collapse'. Getting the fear, and fear based control, out of an organisation can liberate people into imaginative ways of thinking and doing at work that benefit both the organisation and those who make use of its services. So many healthcare settings are ossified by traditional models of militaristic-style management (job titles still have 'officer' in them; employees are organised into hierarchies and lines of control) and rooted in bureaucratic methods that keep things under control in order to maintain stability, prevent the risks of change and keep litigation at bay. In such organisations, relationships are often fraught, functional, and governed by issues of power and control. Hugman's (1991) thesis explores professional relationships and sees them as having very little to do with making life better for patients and much more to do with keeping people in their place. At all levels of such organisations, the tensions and stresses damage all the players in the game to some degree.

There are many signs that such approaches are evolving into new methods which seek to empower and support people in the workplace, and to build new teams as part of the whole which foster the energy and enterprise of the workforce. This is being done primarily by revisiting the relationships between people and exploring how these can reinvigorate both individuals and the organisations they work in. Many people are very successful at running organisations and/or making lots of money, then die prematurely from stress-related illnesses. 'Addictive behaviour displayed by highly stressed executives takes a huge toll on human life and economically. What multinationals are learning is that if they focus more on relationships and values ... then the expansion of happiness would translate into economic terms too' says Chopra (cited in Simpson 1996) again. According to Chopra, companies such as Starbuck's Coffee, Time Warner and Sony Entertainment are taking spirituality more seriously in the USA, where he 'recently convinced executives within International Creative Management in Hollywood to take periodic retreats, practise meditation and as a result of that embrace spiritual principles'.

A sense of purpose and the need for spiritual values seems to be a message that is getting through to more and more businesses. The Social Venture Network (SVN) is a large and increasing gathering of businesses with strong spiritual, social and environmental commitments. It includes organisations such as The Body Shop and the Danish Bank SBN. The SVN began in the USA over 10 years ago and a European branch now has over 150 members. Simpson (1996) describes the spiritual principles of one member of the SVN being applied in practice. The Auchan group, a major food distributor in France, owned a hypermarket in le Havre which was suffering from high incidences of violence and theft. Auchan could have left the area and cut its losses, but instead, it looked at ways in which it could build more positive relationships with the community, began to employ vandals as security guards, thieves as salespeople and so on, and started a campaign to support neighbourhood activities and community organisations. The project worked. Developing right relationship restored a sense of connection with the local community, brought new meaning and purpose to the enterprise, and improved profits as well. It demonstrated that professional people can live out their spiritual values in their daily lives, and transform relationships and the world around them as a result. Organisations espousing similar spiritual values for the workplace, and often embracing healthcare goals, have multiplied such as the well-established Findhorn Foundation Community in Scotland, Planetree in the USA and the Greenleaf Centre for Servant Leadership in England. These, and many more, share many common aims: a desire to bring spiritual values of cooperation, right relationship, collaboration and meaning into all aspects of their activities, whether health or business.

The Findhorn Foundation (1998), for example, has developed ethical business practices that take account of the ecological crisis, new models of community living and ways of integrating non-denominational spiritual practices such as meditation, Taizé singing and sacred dance (see Chapter 4 for more details) into the everyday pattern of the community. Furthermore, it has sought, through its teaching programmes, conferences and many networks, to encourage holistic healing practices, and the development of its community spiritual principles, in other settings.

The Greenleaf Centre in the UK has modelled its work on the American Quaker, Robert Greenleaf. Greenleaf's philosophy of servant leadership is deeply embedded in the spiritual beliefs and practices of the Quakers, with an emphasis on community action, shared power, devolved governance and justice and fairness in relationships. The members of the Quaker movement have a long and honourable history of 'walking their talk', from the great philanthropist families of Rowntree and Cadbury to the 19th-century prison nurse and missionary Elizabeth Fry, and on to playing a leading role in the recent international campaign to ban landmines. The servant leadership concept seeks to encourage organisations to turn away from leadership styles of 'tired old hierarchical, top down, power in the hands of the few "drive it through" approaches to management and leadership' (Spears 1998). Instead, it offers a vision of organisations whose structures and systems are designed to create places of support where people are trusted to do good work and where the leader is not just a 'boss', but a coach or servant. It emphasises increased service to others, a holistic approach to work and the promotion of a sense of community through power sharing. Such an emphasis on getting the relationships right in the organisation first, by moving away from old hierarchical power structures, is echoed in the healthcare sphere by others such as Wright (1998) and Pearson (1992).

Planetree (Moore 1995) was established in the USA as a non-profit making organisation with the aim of humanising hospitals and demystifying healthcare for patients and their families. Some of the focus is on producing more hospitable environments, a subject we will deal with in more detail in Chapter 4, but the organisation also focuses on developing relationships that foster caring for carers as well as patients. Many hospitals in the USA have signed up to Planetree's programmes and others in the UK are following suit. The programmes may involve anything from patient education to rethinking the structure and decor of a building, from reorganising working patterns to offering complementary therapies. This theme is also replicated in the work of centres such as the Bristol Cancer Help Centre and the Glasgow Homeopathic Hospital. Both of these have striven not only to offer alternatives to conventional therapies, but also to work with staff and patients where both are treated with respect, and environment and culture are nourished. Countless other centres for complementary care, healing and healthcare management have mushroomed around the world along similar lines in the past 20 years. All of these have an emphasis on recognising spiritual principles of cooperation, companionship, holism and healing, where there is a search for meaning and connection.

There are signs that such approaches are beginning to enter the consciousness of mainstream healthcare organisations more widely. Recent policy developments in the NHS, for example, have focused much more on 'clinical governance' – the notion of bringing groups of staff together at clinical level and empowering them to make the decisions that affect their daily work

– rather than relying upon a bureaucratic hierarchy. More medical and nursing schools are developing joint appointments or lecturer-practitioners (Lathlean & Vaughan 1994). Only 10 years ago, hostility to the complementary therapies among orthodox medical practitioners was almost universal. Now, over one-third of general practitioners are prepared to include complementary therapies in their care, and their use has been taken up widely in hospitals (Woodham & Peters 1998). A recent project under the leadership of the Prince of Wales (Foundation for Integrated Medicine 1997) sought to bring together the opposites of the orthodox and complementary practitioner fields. In promoting not 'either/or' but integration, a significant breakthrough has been established in defusing the long standing confrontation between the two camps. It also recognised the need to re-examine the context of much of healthcare if it is to be truly holistic, and to take account of the spirituality of both patients and practitioners. Likewise, the 'medical marriage' approach taken at Findhorn (Featherstone & Forsyth 1997), through its series of publications, conferences and workshops, has made considerable efforts to bring the two views together and promote cooperation and integration. Integration seems to have become the key to opening new doors of informed debate and a more positive rapprochement, and it has been taken up at national government policy levels and in the NHS development plans as well.

Healthcare has also been influenced by policy documents such as patients' charters, emphasising that named professionals should have responsibility for specific patients, especially in the field of nursing (Wright 1993). In response to patients' charters, some organisations have sought to recognise and develop the rights and responsibilities of staff as well, and integrate these into a more humane and caring organisational culture. Some more enlightened employers are demonstrating that they are willing and able to create the type of workplace that is welcoming to both the heart and the soul of the worker. By rooting the often esoteric in practice, a real and significant change can take place in a healthcare institution. A happy workforce is a healthy one, and this reduces both the amount of sick pay required and the problems of absenteeism and inefficiency.

I saw it very much as my job, as the manager of this place, to reduce costs and make it more efficient. But I can't do that just by telling people what to do, or to be nice to each other, or being the macho man. It just doesn't work that way. I am very clear that I have responsibilities to patients, but I have responsibilities to staff too. It's not a case of one or the other, it's both. I can't spend money on patients and ignore the staff, and vice versa. The two are indivisible to me, both sides of the same coin. Apart from the money, there are other good reasons for producing a staff-friendly culture, and those are moral ones. I need to do right by the staff not just because it makes a more efficient service and saves money, but just because it's the humane and right thing to do. My actions are morally driven. I don't have particularly strong religious beliefs, but its part of my whole make up that I should treat others as I would like to be treated. And that means having some power and control over my working practices, being involved in decisions that affect me, being treated with kindness, respect, fairness and honesty. Such an environment to work in brings 'value-added caring'. It may take some effort, but it means I practice what I preach, and the benefits to the people who work here and the patients who use it are enormous.

The approach of the leader-manager to her job may define the whole culture of the workplace. As one study indicated (McClure et al 1983), when those in such positions create organisations where staff feel in right relationship, there are benefits to everyone involved. The better places seem to be where:

... staff nurses state that their leaders are visible in the institution for support and problem resolution. Nurse administrators – both top and middle managers – make rounds on patient units, stop to talk to nurses, discuss patients and nursing problems, and listen attentively and respond to what nurses say. Nurses feel free to discuss their concerns with these administrators, whether they relate to patient care, administration, interpersonal relationships or personal matters. They know that their administrators care and that the staff's opinions are valued. (McClure et al 1983).

Recognising the failure of many organisations to care for their carers, the National Association of Staff Support (NASS 1992) developed a staff charter which provided a stimulus for many settings to do likewise. The charter emphasises a wide range of staff rights, such as protection from violence in the workplace, participation in decision-making, personal and professional support, and the freedom of staff to act upon their conscience. The notion of rights was also, interestingly, backed up with comments on the responsibilities of staff, such as giving support to colleagues, keeping their practices up to date and giving loyal service in return. The notion here is of a right relationship that is not one way, but where each works with the other in mutual support, valuing each other's roles. Snow & Willard's study (1989) made recommendations, some of them similar to the work of NASS, including access to collaborative governance at work, access to a male or female counsellor, the right to change values and practices at work 'which seek to shame or devalue me'; the right to 'be respected for the individual I am'; the right to 'my own sacred ground' (such as opportunities for quietness and relaxation at work, time to be alone and reflect, privacy and confidentiality, having one's beliefs and values' respected) and so on. Once again we see common themes emerging: the significance of right relationship in producing a climate that cares for carers in parallel with patients, which is spiritually inspiring as well as efficient and effective.

While many organisations have a long way to go to develop such a climate at work, many others which have made a start give us cause for optimism. If nothing else, concerns about the costs of staff sickness and absenteeism appear to have goaded some employers into action. Some health trusts are showing signs of developing integrated strategies for the health and wellbeing of their employees, and Janet Snell's (1998) report cites Aintree Hospitals Trust and Frenchay Healthcare Trust as examples where action is being taken. Strategies vary from employing teams of complementary therapists to creating a staff gymnasium, from training managers in health and safety at work to introducing team briefing. Such advances are occurring because of growing awareness of the costs of sickness, absence and staff turnover. A further factor appears to be growing fears by employers of litigation, where employees now find the courts are proving to be increasingly sympathetic in awarding compensation against employers whose staff have suffered ill-health through employment-induced stress (O'Dowd 1998). Perhaps there are some who also see caring for their staff as a moral and humanitarian issue as well.

A recent report from the Health Education Authority (1998) tellingly titled *More than Brown Bread and Aerobics*, has shown how an organisation, the British NHS, dedicated to the health of the nation, has itself a very poor track record in caring for the health of its staff. The costs of sickness and absenteeism to the service are enormous (higher than in private industry), but improving staff health through better sickness 'counselling' (often seen by staff as a disciplinary rather than a supportive measure), or offering access to aerobics or aromatherapy sessions, are seen as inadequate in themselves. What is seen as necessary is a root and branch reappraisal of the managerial culture and a coordinated managerial strategy to tackle staff health problems.

A discernible shift in attitudes by employers seems to be taking place. Apart from the examples mentioned above, we have worked with several organisations that are seeking ways forward. These include:

- A hospital trust which developed a staff development programme available to every member of staff regardless of grade or occupation. It included a succession planning programme and shadowing of staff across departments so that all could understand the workings of the whole team.
- A 'caring for the carers' project in one hospital and community trust, incorporating the building of a labyrinth in the hospital grounds, a meditation and relaxation training programme, team building, attitude surveys, the provision of a staff sanctuary as a quiet place for meditation and relaxation, a counselling service, workload reviews and so on. (See Chapter 4 for more details on these techniques.)
- A private hospital which removed temporary and short-term contracts to give staff a sense of security, and included a right to voice complaints in its staff contracts.
- A unit which developed an anti-bullying and equal opportunities strategy.
- A hospice where shared governance was introduced, an education programme with appropriate access points for all staff, a complementary therapies regime available to staff and patients.
- A unit with a clinical leaders' development programme, learning sets, support for practice development projects, devolved leadership to clinical level, and team building workshops for all levels of staff in mixed groups.

These are a few examples from our recent experience, and we will illustrate them in more depth in the next chapter. They show that, with commitment, it is possible for people in the most ordinary settings to transform their working climate and practices, to create environments where the spiritual needs of staff and patients are taken into account, and to acknowledge the presence of the sacred in the workplace.

RIGHT RELATIONSHIP IN TEAMS

In considering this section, we have been reminded of an old joke that has something to say about teamwork. It refers to the Lone Ranger and his Indian companion, Tonto. Both are cornered by hostile Apaches in a canyon, with seemingly no way out. The Lone Ranger looks at Tonto and says 'Well, my faithful friend, it looks like we've had it this time.' To which Tonto replies 'What's all this "we", paleface?'

This kind of response sums up what many experience in clinical teams: the feelings of inequality in relationships, that colleagues will not back you up when the 'chips are down', that there seems to be more interest in power struggles than collegiality. Hugman's thesis (1991) on the nature of power in the caring professions suggests that, in most instances, professional relationships may not always have the best interests of the patients at heart; rather there is enormous investment of time and energy in subtle, and sometimes not so subtle, struggles for control and authority over others.

> The multidisciplinary team at the clinic is a myth. Everyone gets on reasonably well, we meet and discuss patients at case conferences and everyone has a chance to be heard. But the whole set-up is essentially patronising. The doctor still sees himself as the natural captain of the team, and his attitude is one of 'we're all in the same game together as equals', but underneath that everyone knows that the reality is that he sees himself as the one in overall charge, and if we didn't play the game his way, he'd cry 'foul' and take his ball away!

The recent emphasis on clinical governance in the UK at government policy level seeks to move healthcare teams further away from this paradigm. The ideal team would allow each to take a leadership role, depending on who was best equipped to do so in relation to the patients' needs. The reality for the most part is that doctors, usually male, still see this as very much their role, although the situation does seem to be changing as we shall see (Stein et al 1991). Meanwhile, Charles Handy (1994) has compared the average British team in the workplace to that of a rowing crew – a group of people who cannot see where they are going, frantically rowing backwards and being told what to do by the only person who does not know how to row!

> Since I started work at the hospice it's been like a breath of fresh air. The team spirit is unbelievable. Everyone just gets on with their work and helps everyone else. It's a world away from the cancer hospital, with its prima donna professors and posturing matrons, and the scale of staff with everyone neatly slotted into their

place on the ladder. Here there's none of that nonsense. When the doctor arrives he's just as likely to put the kettle on and make us all a cuppa as ask our views on a patient's progress. There's no way that would have happened at my last job. Hospitality was definitely something that we were expected to provide as soon as the 'gods' arrived on the wards. It's not just the tea thing though, it's the whole atmosphere of the place. There's a sense of us all being in this together, of pulling in the same direction. And I think that helps the patients too. There's no 'us and them', just a lot of us in the same place trying to solve a lot of problems together.

Faugier (1996) believes that 'one of the most important lessons for all of us is that the resolution of interdisciplinary conflict enables us to take a combined look at the most important interface – the relationship with those who use the service'. By transforming the way we work together, we can thereby transform the way we work with patients. Relationships, right relationships, in teams that have meaning and purpose for us and which satisfies the need in each of us to feel connected, respected and valued as a human being and contributor to the team, need working at; they take practice and constant re-examination and maintenance if they are to keep working well. Historically, in the business world and in many healthcare organisations, it has been custom and practice for those at the top of the organisation to take time out, sabbaticals, team-building weekends and so on. Those who work at the clinical level, who actually do the caring, rarely have such opportunities. In part, this is because of the sheer logistics of arranging such events. Everyone could not leave at once, or who would look after the patients? The idea may sound fine in principal, but in practice there is often little allowance of time or funding for such events to be created for the 'hands-on' carers. This may seem a peculiar reversal of values. After all, as far as patients are concerned, who is most important to them? Who is it that they depend upon to be most effective in their job? Not the director of finance. Not the head of human resources. Not the chief executive. It is the nurses, doctors and other therapists and healers who are of priority to patients. That is not to say that those other roles are not important; they are, but the service deliverers need opportunities for effective teamwork and team building too.

Employees in an organisation that has grasped the principles of servant leadership, clinical governance and empowerment of staff have no problem understanding the significance of clinical teams and of fostering their development. As suggested in the previous section, the organisational culture itself needs to shift to encourage the growth of right relationship in teams. Once this process is under way, then the teams can begin to reappraise the ways in which they work together.

We organised a team away weekend with plenty of notice and almost everyone got to it. To cover the unit, the managers came in and took charge and brought in extra staff on overtime. I found that alone to be impressive. I really didn't believe it until it actually happened. The first morning was the most difficult. We did an 'unmasking' exercise with the help of the facilitator. We had to talk about who we really are, our hopes, our dreams, our struggles, our families, our histories. I don't think one of us in that room found it easy to stop being physiotherapist, or doctor, or nurse or whoever. Of course what dawned on me after a little while was 'My God, these people are just like me!' It seems odd to say it like that. Some of these people I'd worked with for years. I knew lots about them, or thought I did, but something else happened that morning – I 'felt' for them, I felt like I was getting to know them for the first time. The effects have stayed with me ever since, and none of us has been the same since. That, and all the other things we did that weekend seemed to produce a greater sense of trust between each other. After it, we seemed to respond to each other in so many more positive ways. We still have our roles to play, but I know now that's not the real person, not who they really are. Even when things are fraught, we seem to pull together rather than start bickering with and blaming each other. There seems to be so much more respect around between us, so much more, dare I say it, Love? (Figure 3.1)

Participating in groups like this can be a joyous and a painful experience. Letting go of who we think we are, and who we think others are, is no easy task. It means that we have to admit to being less than in control, that we are not 'supercarer' who can manage anything. It means we have to look at our uncertainties, our frailties, our tragedies, as well as the parts of ourselves where there is certainty, strength and joy. Where teams of people commit themselves to this kind of work and are supported in doing so, then the possibility of right relationship emerging or being strengthened opens up before them. Furthermore, building effective teams does not just rely upon

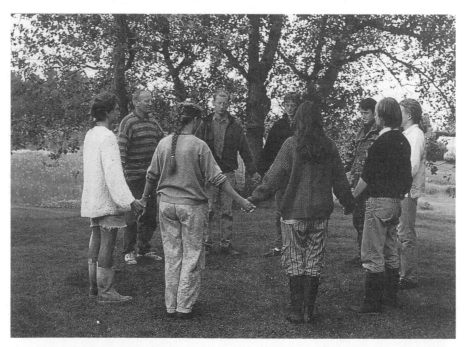

Figure 3.1 Coming together to refocus how we work as a team affects everything we do in the working day or night. © Forder & Forder, reprinted with permission.

time out from work with expert facilitators. Other aspects of work can make a contribution, for example:

- setting up shared educational programmes, study days, seminars and workshops for carers from all backgrounds
- working as part of a multidisciplinary project group
- working together to set up protocols and joint guidance to help us share work or become clearer about areas where boundaries overlap.
- organising regular social events
- using group clinical supervision of a multidisciplinary nature to explore common boundaries, problems and issues of practice development.
- identifying clearly what our roles are and what is expected of each other in our working relationships.
- making away-days, team-building exercises and other such events a regular part of the team's calendar, rather than one-off events
- networking with other groups with similar interests
- setting up a networking newsletter for the whole team
- setting up pre- and post-shift group debriefing sessions
- providing sessions in meditation, relaxation techniques, assertiveness, stress management or T'ai chi, for example
- introducing 'quiet space' on the unit, e.g. time set aside when all activity is reduced to a minimum for at least an hour each afternoon, for the benefit of both staff and patients.

These are some points that we have observed with various groups in the past few years. One multidisciplinary group known to us took Marie Manthey's (1982) 'Commitment to Each Other' statement and worked with this to re-evaluate the way they were working together. Eventually, they produced a collaborative statement which included comments such as 'I will be committed to finding solutions to problems, rather than complaining about them or blaming someone for them, and ask you to do the same' and 'I will establish and maintain a relationship with you and every member of the staff. My relationships with each of you will be equally respectful, regardless of job titles or levels of educational preparation'. Six other points on similar themes about right relationship were included in the full statement.

Another group (Findhorn Foundation 1998) took up the suggestion of Caroline Myss, a widely published healer noted among other things for her intuitive diagnostic abilities, to create a code of conduct. The community worked on and developed such statements as 'I commit myself to active spiritual practice and to align with spirit to work the greatest good', and 'I commit myself to the service of others and to our planet, recognising that I must also serve myself in order to practise effectively' and 'I commit wholeheartedly to respect other people (their differences, their views, their origins, backgrounds and issues)' and so on, some 14 statements being agreed in all.

There are several key points to note about statements like these. First, they are made by groups themselves coming together and agreeing and stating openly what feels right for them. They are not produced by management edict or dominant group members. Second, they are used: they are living documents, available to guide people if a conflict emerges, to help new team members and so on. Third, the process people have gone through to produce such statements is probably more important than the written outcome. It is rarely necessary to memorise them or revise them every day. In making the statements, the way people have arrived at the wording and the meaning establishes a common bond of understanding, of shared goals and shared meaning in our day-to-day relationships.

Although many people still work in environments where genuine collegiate relationships have yet to be realised, there are many areas where the shift towards right relationships in teams is taking place. Taking a historical perspective, there is some evidence for this. Stein (1978) discussed the 'doctor–nurse game', where the doctor was always supposed to be superior and in control, and the nurse was always to be deferential while using guile or wily manipulation to get her way in the relationship. Much the same seems to have applied to relationships between healthcare professionals and patients or lay carers. The traditional model holds that patients and informal carers are supposed to be obedient and grateful: once again we see power and control struggles at work at all levels of such relationships. However, it seems that these old stereotypical roles are now less typical in healthcare. Stein and his colleagues (1991), revisiting their original work 13 years later, discovered much more realistic teamwork taking place, driven in part by the feminist movement, changing power structures in healthcare, more women entering medicine, more men entering nursing, and better educated nurses. Perhaps what is taking place in the wider world, the social phenomenon loosely described as the New Age with its personal search for meaning and assertion of personal identity in the world, has had an inevitable knock-on effect on team members in the healthcare setting. They are part of that wider society after all. Each individual's learning, development and spiritual path will influence the wider world. When we want to change things around us, the first step may be to change ourselves inside. It is to the work of the individual that we will now turn.

THE INDIVIDUAL (Fig. 3.2)

One of the effects of the whining and whingeing behaviour discussed in Chapter 1 is that this acts as a kind of self-justification, a self-esteem booster when things around us do not make us feel as good as we might wish. It enables us to see the problems in the organisation or team as other people's fault: 'we are all right really – it is everyone and everything else that is to blame'. Butterworth & Faugier (1994) note how there are two classic responses when groups of healthcare workers get together, be it at a meeting, a

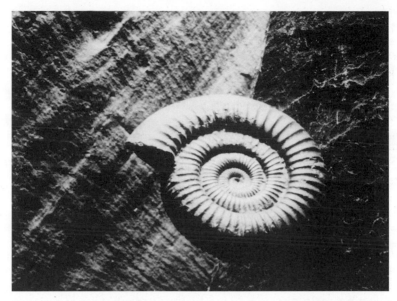

Figure 3.2   The spiral, an archetypal symbol for wholeness in many cultures and symbolic of the individual's journey inward and outward. © Laurence Winram, reprinted with permission.

conference or a social event. There is the 'we are ever so wonderful' response – 'everything out there may be terrible, the managers don't understand us, the patients are always complaining, but that's because they don't appreciate how dedicated and essential we are', and there is the 'we must be mad to work here' response – 'everything about the place of work is terrible, the managers are appalling, the resources inadequate, but we soldier on martyr-like and keep the ship afloat; we must be mad to put up with this and work in such a place'. Both postures, while somewhat amusing, serve to do little more than give a minor boost to our collective and individual self-esteem by assuming that it is really everyone else who is at fault, and both postures also keep us stuck where we are in our victim mentality.

Holding the sacred in the workplace through right relationship demands a collective effort on the part of the wider organisation, every team and every individual. No one part can manage it alone. Frances Vaughan (1995) writes that

'It is up to us, each one of us, to take responsibility for making the changes in our lives that will enable us to contribute to the wellbeing of the whole. If we aspire to optimum health either individually or collectively we must learn to pay attention to all aspects of physical, emotional, mental, existential and spiritual wellbeing'.

When we begin focusing in on ourselves, especially those of us working in healthcare systems and professions that are so obsessed with power, control and defensiveness, we can begin to change ourselves. This may be at considerable personal sacrifice in terms of time, effort, money and the pain of inner reflection and change, but the impact on patient care in the long term may be profound.

> I reached the age of 40 before I began to wake up to what might be called my spiritual journey. Over the next 5 or 6 years, I began the search in earnest, I meditated, I returned to church, I read spiritual texts obsessively, I went on workshops and courses to get more insight into myself. I worked with a psychotherapist for 2 years to see what was going on in me. It was an astonishing, surprising, exciting, painful, difficult, wonderful time, and it's still going on. I have learned much from it, not least that I can change, that things that used to really hurt can be let go, that in changing myself in so many ways, people notice the difference after a while … 'you're less easily upset' they say, or 'you're easier to be around' or 'you don't seem as distracted when I talk to you' … things like that. This way, I think, I am making a difference in some subtle way to the way the whole team works together. If by working a little one can have that kind of impact, then I wonder what would happen if 5, 10, 15 percent of the staff here began to shift like me … we could change the world!

Our spiritual work and our personal, emotional work are closely connected. It is not possible to bypass the latter and leap straight to the former. There are no short cuts. Personal development is about taking responsibility, being self-reliant, setting goals, discovering our history and what life experiences have made us who we are today. Spiritual development concerns self-observation, contemplation and/or meditation plus moderation of the ego, not feeling that you have to fill your life with material status symbols, and letting go of jealousy and envy. 'When you stop worrying about pleasing and impressing others, you start to grow spiritually' (Turner 1996). However, the task of spiritual development is by no means an easy one. One session sitting cross legged on the floor is unlikely to project us instantly to inner truth: it takes time to confront and deal with the fears that block the path to intimacy with overselves.

If the heart of spirituality is relationships – with each other, ourselves, our environment and the beyond – then perhaps it is in relationships that we can experience the sacred:

… impediments to intimacy in our lives are also barriers to spirituality. Giving ourselves to someone or something beyond ourselves requires trust and surrender. We fear trust and surrender because they appear to threaten us with the loss of ourself. Thus meaning and intimacy both come hard to us, if they come at all. (Jones 1996)

Learning to trust each other is a significant factor in producing right relationships in teams and organisations, and with those we care for. That trust is all the more difficult to achieve unless we have learned to trust our deepest selves. And yet, as Jones goes on to point out, 'We must develop a strong sense of self before we can give that self away, but it is only on giving the self away that we finally find our self'. In other words, who we think we are must be discovered and surrendered, in order to find out who we really are. 'Our goal', as Carey (1991) points out, 'is not to end individuality, but to inhabit it'. Who we think we are is but a transient persona constructed to serve us in this reality, it is not the eternal transcendent core that is our real identity. But to discover it, that is the difficulty; it takes hard work. Spirituality is both a theory and a practice. The word 'experiment' and 'experience' have the same origin. If we carry out certain actions, we may expect to experience a connection with the sacred, and when that happens, we may find ourselves able to bring that experience back into the world in new and fulfilling ways that not only transform our own world, but that of those around us. To find the place within each of us where the sacred dwells, we must be willing to open ourselves to undertake the journey, and this spiritual journey does not just consist of experiences of light and bliss, as we shall see in Chapter 5. Deciding to make the journey is the most important first step, although for some people, making a decision to pursue a spiritual path may be beyond choice. Triggered by life's events, it may take on a momentum of its own that may seem all but impossible to stop, where there seems little choice but to go on.

There is an old Hindu story about an argument between the gods about where to hide the secret of life and happiness from people. 'Put it in the deepest, darkest forest' said one, 'they will never find it there'. 'No,' said another, 'they will one day cut the trees down and discover it'. 'Hide it at the bottom of the ocean,' said one, 'No,' said another, 'one day they will learn to swim the deeps and reach our secret'. 'I know,' said the goddess, place it in men's hearts, they will never think of looking there'. And so it was that the secret of life and happiness has been hidden from us ever since. The path with heart is our route to understanding who we are, the sacred within ourselves. Once discovered, we may bring all that it contains out into the world. Barbara Graham (1995) writes that 'The path that leads us to a reality greater than ourselves inevitably, paradoxically, twists and spirals downward to the self, where God, Love, our Buddha nature … are all right there, smiling, waiting for us to come home.'

Frank Ashton, a counsellor and therapist who we have worked with in healthcare team building and personal development, often starts a group session with a series of simple questions. It is not meant to be taken terribly seriously, just to act as a key to unlock the door to insight within each of us. Illness for anyone can be a stew of panic, fear, pain, anger and denial. In such a stew, we as carers need to be well grounded in ourselves if we are not to be caught up in co-dependence, which can lead to exhaustion and burnout. Checking out how well we take care of ourselves can be a good starting point for asking deeper questions about our own inner journey. Try answering the following questions, yes or no (treat a 'maybe' as a 'no'). We suggest that you do not think about the questions too much, just accept the answer that first comes to you – it's probably the most accurate! Do you:

1. have what you regard as regular sleep habits?
2. eat a healthy diet?
3. take plenty of exercise?

4. talk through problems with a partner/close friend?
5. talk through problems with colleagues?
6. talk through problems with your boss?
7. practise meditation or relaxation?
8. withdraw from stressful situations appropriately?
9. set aside one day each month to do exactly as you please?
10. allow yourself a good read or something similar, every day, for at least half an hour, that takes all of your attention and is nothing to do with work?
11. give yourself breaks and treats when you need them?
12. practise being quiet and avoiding the centre of attention?

Any score of 6 'yes's' or less may mean that you have a problem with stress and anxiety at work. Score 7–11, and you appear to be taking care of yourself, but there's no room for complacency and you may indeed be in denial! Score 12, and you're probably not being truthful!

The purpose of this simple exercise is to encourage us to think about how we take care of ourselves, and perhaps begin the first steps through insight about how we might make life a little less fraught. Taking care of ourselves may be the first tentative step to a longer journey of self-discovery that eventually leads us home. Alternatively, the questions may do nothing more than stimulate us to try one or two things to look after ourselves better, for example, looking at our diet, increasing our exercise levels or seeking clinical supervision. This short questionnaire is not an attempt to make people feel guilty because they have not achieved a high score; indeed the questions are open to some degree of interpretation, but they do give us some clues about where we might start to look to make that long journey of the path to the inner self. In each question, there is also a suggestion for a way we can take care of ourselves: the more we can find time for, the more we will benefit.

In the next chapter, we will look in a little more detail about what some of these steps might be, the tools to aid us in our spiritual journey. If we commit ourselves to undertaking the journey, the possibilities are boundless. We may come to realise and affirm what was said in the Introduction, that sacred space is not something 'out there' but also 'in here'. Janet Quinn (1992) reminds us of this potential:

'No one and no thing can heal another human being. All healing is creative emergence, new birth, the manifestation of the powerful inner longing to be whole'.

In the spirit of 'physician heal thyself', we find a repeating echo: look to ourselves first; become centred and clear in who we are and why we are here; learn to trust and let go; heal our own wounds; discover who we really are; come home to ourselves. Then, as Quinn goes on to say,

'We can remove barriers to the healing process (Plate 5). We can participate in creating healing environments that will support healing. We can become midwives to the process of healing, creating and being safe sacred space into which the healing might emerge. We can, literally, become the healing environment'.

Shifting the organisation and the team to a spiritual focus in our work depends also on our own spiritual path. Without a concerted effort in all these directions, we may be but tinkering at the edges in our efforts to create and hold healing environments in which the sense of the sacred pervades every living moment. Such a process begins and ends with ourselves. Becoming aware, not just of what we do, but of the significance of who we are allows us to become the very healing environment, the present and available carer in whom caring is effortless because it comes not from the shallow trough of our own egos and personalities, but from the deep well of our true being, the sacred centre, expressed in every caring moment. It is not so much what we do that heals; it is who we are.

Thus strengthened, we can enter the caring milieu wherever we find it – in the home, the hospice, the hospital, the clinic, the office, the factory or wherever caring is needed. We are the sacred space: it lives in us, and is held all around us. It starts within us, and once searched for, found and nourished, we can bring it into the wider world, transforming organisations, teams, situations and events from within. The only thing that holds us back is fear. We may dress it up with reasons or excuses, but when the mask is removed, there it is: fear. In Chapter 4, we will discuss how we can learn to overcome some of this fear and bring right relationship and the sacred into our everyday lives.

REFERENCES

Adams P 1993 Gezundheit. Healing Arts Press, Rochester NJ
Buber M 1937 I and thou. Clarke, Edinburgh
Butterworth A, Faugier J 1994 Clinical supervision in nursing, midwifery and health visiting – a briefing paper. School of Nursing Studies, University of Manchester
Carey K 1991 The third millenium. Harper, San Francisco
Chopra D 1996 The seven spiritual laws of success. Bantam, London
Faugier J 1996 Unhealthy relations. Nursing Times 11 (92):50
Featherstone C, Forsyth L 1997 The medical marriage. Findhorn Press, Findhorn
Findhorn Foundation 1998 Statement of common ground. Findhorn Foundation, Findhorn
Foundation for Integrated Medicine 1997 Integrated healthcare. FIM, London
Goleman D 1995 Emotional intelligence. Bantam, New York
Graham B 1995 Looking for love in all the wrong places. Common Boundary Sept/Oct: 71–72
Health Education Authority 1998 More than brown bread and aerobics. HEA, London
Jones J 1996 In the middle of this road we call our life. HarperCollins, London
Handy C 1994 The empty raincoat. Arrow, Sydney
Hatfield D 1999 Gallup Organisation: New research links emotional intelligence with profitability. The Inner Edge 1(5): 5–9
Hugman R 1991 Power in caring professions. Macmillan, London
Lathlean J, Vaughan B 1994 Unifying nursing practice and theory. Butterworth-Heinemann, Oxford
Manthey M 1982 A commitment to each other. Cited in Wright S G 1993 My patient – my nurse. Scutari, Harrow
McClure M L, Puolin M A, Sovie M D, Wandelt M A 1983 Magnet hospitals – attraction and retention of professional nurses. American Academy of Nursing, Kansas

Moore N 1995 Planetree: changing the way we think about patients. Alternative Therapies in Health and Medicine 1(1): 14

National Association for Staff Support 1992 A charter for staff support. NASS, Woking

O'Dowd A 1998 Courting disaster. Nursing Times 94(37): 16–17

Pearson A 1992 Burford – a story of change. Scutari, Harrow

Quinn J 1992 Holding sacred space: the nurse as healing environment. Holistic Nursing Practice 6(4): 26–36

Simpson L 1996 Principles and profits. Business News June: 26–30

Snell J 1998 Saying it with flowers. Health Service Journal, August: 21–23

Snow C, Willard P 1989 I'm dying to take care of you. Professional Counseller Books, Redmond

Spears L C (ed) 1998 Insights on leadership – service, stewardship, spirit and servant leadership. London, Wiley

Stein L 1978 The doctor – nurse game. In: Dingwall R, MacIntosh J 1978 Readings in the Sociology of Nursing. Churchill Livingstone, Edinburgh

Stein L, Watts D, Howell T, 1991 The doctor – nurse game revisited. New England Journal of Medicine 322(8): 546–549

Toms M 1999 Emotional intelligence in the workplace: an interview with Daniel Goleman. The Inner Edge 1(5): 14–17

Turner C 1996 The eureka principle. Element, London

Vaughan F 1995 Shadows of the sacred. Quest, Wheaton

Woodham A, Peters D 1998 The encyclopaedia of complementary medicine. Dorling Kindersley, London

Wright S G 1993 The named nurse, midwife and health visitor. NHSE, Leeds

Wright S G 1998 Changing nursing practice. Arnold, London

PLATE 1

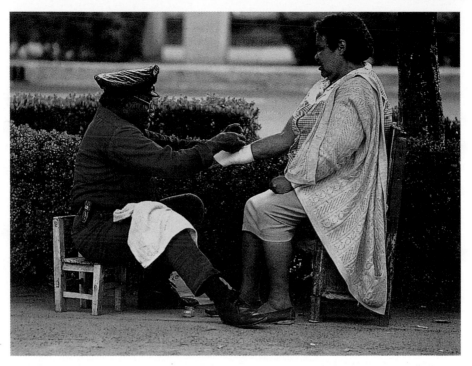

Plate 1 A street healer in Brazil: therapeutic relationships are not exclusive to professionals. © Eric Lars Bakke, reprinted with permission.

PLATE 2

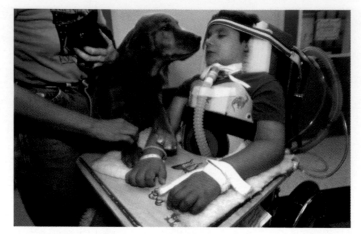

Plate 2 Healing relationships are not just with people and seem to work perfectly well without 'superhood'. © P. F. Bentley 2000, reprinted with permission.

PLATE 3

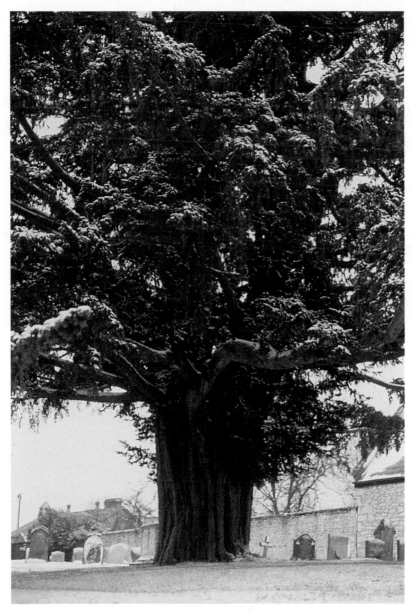

Plate 3   The yew tree, one of the most long-lived of all organisms, sacred to many cultures and often associated with the notion of the whole environment as being part of healing. Yew tree, churchyard of the Blessed Virgin Mary, Batcombe, Somerset. © Cindy A. Pavlinac, reprinted with permission.

PLATE 4

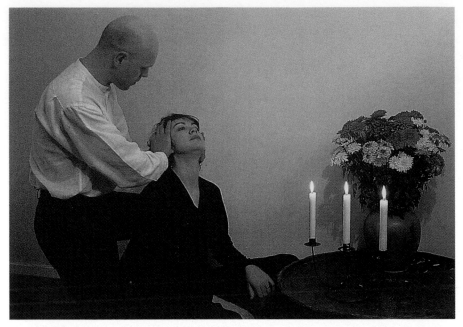

Plate 4 There can be a moment in healing when both are transported to a place of mystery.
© Forder & Forder.

PLATE 5

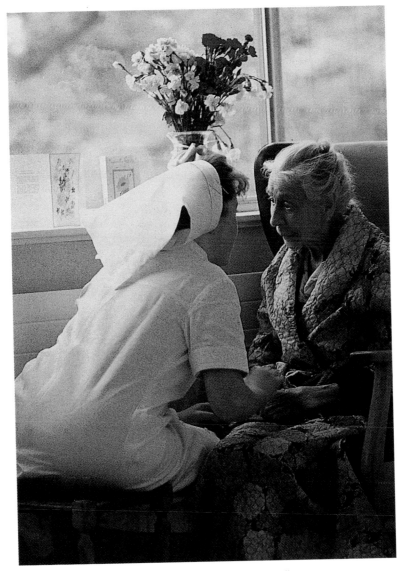

Plate 5 Being who we are, we can remove barriers to the healing process.

PLATE 10

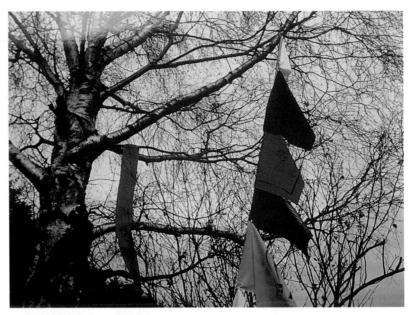

Plate 10   Any place and moment can become sacred if we choose it.

4

Pathways to the sacred

A vision without a task is but a dream.
A task without a vision is drudgery.
A vision and a task are the hope of the world.

Inscription, Sussex Churchyard

OPENING THE GATE

In the previous chapter we suggested three key areas in caring relationships where work can be done to encourage right relationship and nourish sacred space. This chapter gives an overview of a number of pathways to pursue those goals. There are thousands of possibilities, techniques or pathways to choose from, some ancient and some modern. Our selection is governed by our experience – what has worked for us – and other options that are emerging into common use. It is not possible, because of the space available in this book, to give great detail about each one. Our intention is to offer a taste from the vast selection that is on offer, so any that appeal to the reader can then be pursued in greater depth. These various options might best be seen as openings or gateways into an expanded awareness of who we are. The first requirement, having made the discovery of what sounds and feels right, is to take the first steps through: one step into the light is one step out of the dark. It may be that you have already become aware of your journey and chosen a path; if not, we invite you to take that step now.

It is important to be relaxed about choosing a particular path. One that seems irrelevant now may emerge as significant at a later date. Likewise, while we may choose some paths, such as meditation or prayer, as part of a lifetime commitment to deepening our spiritual practice and our appreciation of the sacred, we may find that some things run their course and we then wish to let go of them. There is no point in pursuing a particular method just for the sake of it, or because we feel guilty for not keeping it going. However, this has to be balanced with the commitment to making the effort, especially through the difficult phases which inevitably occur. That may be the point at which we need to be most resolute in order to gain the benefits that lie beyond.

It is vital to be very clear about our motives for choosing a particular path. Do we want to be more centred in ourselves so that we can be more effective in caring, be of service, find deeper meaning and purpose in life, perhaps God? Or do we wish to increase our sense of power and control over others, to engage in spiritual one-upmanship – 'I am more enlightened than you are!' Spending some time seeking guidance from a trusted friend, counsellor or teacher may help us to become clearer not just about where we want to go, but why. We see little purpose in taking up meditation, for example, if our intent is to strengthen our power over others or drop out from worldly concerns completely. In fact, to pursue these avenues for self-gratification can be very dangerous: we fail to become more spiritually aware and available to others, and instead we simply reinforce the darker side of ourselves, our frustrations and neuroses. The paths we recommend all have one central goal in common: to deepen awareness of ourselves, so that we can be of service in the world more effectively, i.e. with less stress, burnout, pain and suffering for ourselves and those around us.

Deepening our understanding of ourselves, we 'come home', enter into right relationship with ourselves, with others and beyond (whatever or whoever we perceive that to be). Hadewijch II, a 13th-century Flemish member of the Beguines – a lay women's movement which created independent spiritual communities across Europe (cited in McLuhan 1996) – wrote:

> You who want knowledge
> seek the Oneness
> within
> There you will find
> the clear mirror
> already waiting.

There are options open to us to look into that 'clear mirror'. Indeed, the apparent 'spiritual supermarket' of choices that exists today, while providing many avenues for self-improvement, can also expose us to the risks of charlatanism and quackery, as will be discussed in Chapter 5. Frances Vaughan (1995) notes that:

Many different spiritual paths are currently available. Among those symbolically portrayed as leading up a mountain, some are hard and narrow, others soft and gentle. Some are more scenic and meandering than others and many seem to spiral into new ways of perceiving reality. All ostensibly lead to a summit of spiritual maturity, described by such terms as enlightenment, salvation or liberation. Other metaphors of spiritual development include escape from captivity followed by a sojourn in the wilderness, winding from the periphery to the center of a labyrinth, or cultivating a garden.

Thus, in this chapter we will consider actual labyrinths and gardens, but they and the other tools we will look at can also be seen as metaphors for something else that may be taking place. When we tend our garden at home, it can be like a meditation, where our attention is so focused afterwards that we can feel relaxed, centred and perhaps have received new insights or resolutions to problems or difficulties that beset us. Likewise, walking a labyrinth can have the same effect. The physical actions we undertake can be a mirror for what is going on internally: tending the garden and its flowers reflects the tending of our own inner garden; walking the labyrinth reflects the inner journey that is going on simultaneously.

The small number of options for spiritual work that we can cover here are only part of a much bigger picture. They may be used as part of an orthodox religious path: it is not necessary to give up an established faith or religious practice. We see the following as adjuncts to that, not distracters. Indeed, it has been our experience that such methods have tended to strengthen people's existing religious roots rather than undermine them. We have, therefore, not looked at this chapter from a perspective of different faiths. It is not our role to recommend a particular religious path; indeed, there may be no need to chop and change or mix and match religions. The chances are that the particular religious and spiritual route that is right for us may be already right under our own noses, embedded in our own life experience and culture.

Furthermore, we have thus far made clear links between our own health and relationships in the caring context and their spiritual underpinnings. What we seek to do here is offer a number of suggestions which may be sought out and applied in the workplace, the home or other community. The aim of each is to deepen our understanding of ourselves, to help us be clearer about what makes us tick and how we are in the world. Each of the following tools has the capacity to help us along that road, to help us to find that place within that has heart and meaning for us. In that sense, all the following are spiritual tools to help us into right relationship with ourselves and thereby our colleagues and those we care for. None of them alone will solve all our problems overnight, bring us instant enlightenment or turn us into perfect human beings. They may, however, nudge us that little bit further along our own unique spiritual journey, helping to transform the way in which we care for ourselves and others. Strengthening right relationship in our caring roles, we become more aware of the sacred space that is present.

THE CARING ENVIRONMENT

So much of the caring context of the modern world, be it the home or the hospital, has seen the sacred sacrificed to functionalism. In the near obsession to be clean and prevent infection, to have buildings that can be cheaply built and easily managed, and in an effort to avoid any particular religious symbolism that might offend one party or another, we have birthed environments where people often recover from sickness in spite of, rather than because of them. Mann (1993) believes that modern architecture has lost its way, and an indicator is how few architects actually live in the buildings they create. He believes that:

... the sacred lives in buildings or monuments in which the structure and decoration follow clear and basic patterns derived from the ancient conception of the four elements, earth, water, air and fire, the forms of nature and from living energies and the geometries derived from them. Proportion systems, amplifying natural rhythms and patterns bring a natural and organic energy and spirituality to sacred architecture – the building contains an elemental as well as human quality evoking the spiritual.

So little of modern architecture, of home or institution, seems to reflect the human or elemental.

We were determined that this time it would be different, that the new hospital would be as much a part of the patients' healing as the staff and the treatments. We began the planning looking at the principles of sacred geometry and sacred space, how to make the building and its proportions on a scale that would be harmonious with people and that would create a feeling of welcome and wellbeing. We invited present and former patients along to the foundation-laying ceremony, and we plan to have a garden that will not only be aesthetically pleasing, but which will also provide organic food for the kitchen.

Replacing the often inhuman buildings used for healthcare will take generations (Figure 4.1) New buildings – hospitals and clinics – are being constructed as this is written which, while notionally places of healing, will turn out to be anything but. It is true that relationships, as we have stressed throughout this text, are more important in many respects than what people do or where they work, but the context can profoundly affect these factors, except for all but the most centred and spiritually awake human beings. Many of us do not even notice the effects the environment may be having on

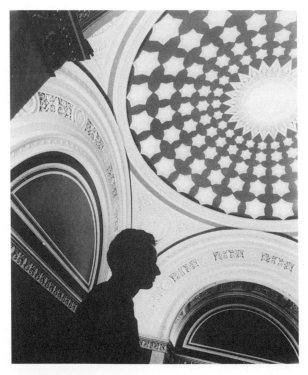

Figure 4.1 Sacred architecture: the building can be as much a part of the healing as any treatment. © Laurence Winram, reprinted with permission.

us, we just get so used to working in those conditions that we fail to see how they may be hostile to the way we work or how they affect the way we feel. We may notice the difference only when someone comes along and makes some changes, such as redesigning a garden or the decor of a unit.

Some places and people are, however, giving a lead on these issues – not least the Prince of Wales' committees and advisers on sacred architecture, and the School of Architecture at the University of Humberside. Many new building projects are showing a responsiveness to sacred aesthetics as well as to function, and this has especially been the case in the hospice movement and centres for complementary care such as those in Eskdale and Bristol, or the retreat facilities for health workers at the Sacred Space Foundation.

Interestingly, the need for the sacred in the physical environment is not a new idea (Figure 4.2). Whether people have created certain special sacred places, or merely discovered that which is already there and built upon them, is open to debate. For millennia, people have sought to identify and work with certain places where healing, ritual, ceremony and so on could be gathered and held. From the stone circles, pyramids, symbolic sites and neolithic tombs of ancient peoples across the world, to modern cathedrals or ceremonial places, we seem to have always sought to either construct or be among places where we can feel, if only for a moment, the healing and peace that comes with a sense of the transcendent, of being part of something other than

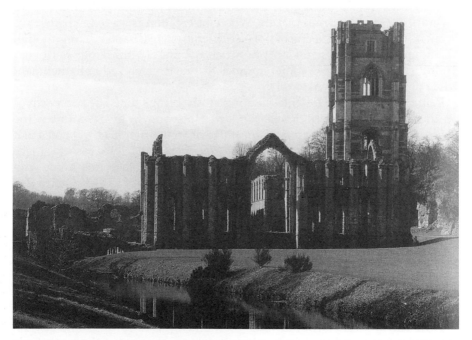

Figure 4.2 Many sacred places were also designed as places of healing: Fountains Abbey, Yorkshire. © Forder & Forder, reprinted with permission.

ourselves, of union with some force or power, whatever we have named it, that makes us feel whole. Indeed, the words 'healing' and 'whole' are derived from the same linguistic roots.

Whether we have built places to attune us to the spirit (McLuhan 1996, Palmer & Palmer 1997) or whether we have found 'soul food' in places that are natural and relatively untouched by people, the effect is the same. Some can find as much of a spiritual quality in the hills and valleys of the Lake District of England as in their back garden or local church (Forder & Forder 1995), in the magnificence of Monument Valley in the American Southwest or under an ancient yew tree in a remote part of Scotland (Chetan & Brueton 1994, Pakenham 1996), in a great forest or looking at a plant in the living room. We have always found solace, comfort and a sense of 'coming home' or being at one with ourselves in the natural world around us as well as in the constructed. St Bernard of Clairvaux (cited in McLuhan 1996) wrote: 'What I know of the divine sciences and Holy Scripture, I learnt in the woods and fields. I have no other masters than the beeches and the oaks'. McLuhan also quotes the words of the Sufi mystic, Abu Hamid Muhammad al-Ghazzali: 'the visible world was made to correspond to the world invisible and there is nothing in this world but a symbol of something in that world'.

The notion of correspondence, that what we see and feel in this reality corresponds with and can be a reflection to us of that which is internal and invisible, means that when we tune in to what is around us in the everyday world, we may also tune into the transcendent, the sacred (Maxwell & Tschudin 1990). The belief that the whole of creation is sacred, whether we deem it aesthetically pleasing or not (see discussion in Chapter 5) runs though all the great belief systems and in much of modern thinking. A Tibetan Buddhist story reminds us that an ancient master received enlightenment while observing his own excreta!

Palmer & Palmer's (1997) fascinating study brings together perspectives on the sacred from right across the UK. Here and in every country, the landscape is seen as the sacred all around us. Diana Brueton (1997) notes that the word for this in Welsh is *cynefin* – 'the place in which I am at ease, the place I want to be, perhaps even the place of my being'. This place, this 'home', can be anywhere, but it may be that the most important place to feel at home, for which the outer world is but a reflection, is within ourselves. When we enter into right relationship with ourselves, then everywhere is home. Where we are in the outer world may no longer be of significance to us when we are always at home within, and resting in that place, we are immensely more capable of being of service to others without the sense of it being a burden. However, getting to that inner home is aided, for a time at least, by the way we use the environment of the outer world. In being at rest, at home there, we may come to rest more easily in ourselves.

How can we transform our often sterile healthcare settings into *cynefin*, where the heart and soul feel welcome, when so many of those we have created or had created for us have lost this spirit of place. The sacred may be all around, and inside us, but it is much more difficult to see it in the fraught world of a clean-walled casualty department than in a peaceful country churchyard. Many sacred places are spoiled by spiritual tourism – those who come to stand and stare, take photographs, let the children run riot over them, spill their drinks and drop their cigarette ends over them (Pennick 1996). If special sacred sites, with all that they have to teach us, have been so desecrated, how can we possibly hope to bring such influences in to the frantic work world or the busy home? Is it too much to expect to keep up with the demands of caring for another, let alone look to our environment beyond cleanliness and tidiness? What we can do is create new traditions and practices, or revive old ones, in ways appropriate to existing conditions. 'Spirituality has not gone away', despite the circumstances in which we find ourselves: 'it is still there for anyone who seeks it' (Pennick 1996). Thus there may be some traditions and practices that we can now work with to restore a sense of sacred into the caring context.

Architecture

We can review and revisit the principles of sacred architecture with architects, planners and others involved in the construction of buildings to be used for healthcare (and this includes the patients and carers who will occupy them). One example is the joint project with the University of Humberside's School of Architecture and the Sacred Space Foundation to document and disseminate best practice which combines sacred architecture principles with hospital and clinic design. Such an approach would have seemed common sense to Florence Nightingale (1859), who wrote extensively, not only about the nature of the healing nurse–patient relationship, but also about hospital design for good hygiene, light and air in combination with beauty and symmetry. A further good practical example of this approach is the work being undertaken to construct the new homeopathic hospital in Glasgow, where an attempt is being made to involve users at every stage of the creation of the building, to construct a hospital which is as much a part of the healing process as the people who work in it.

The notion of sacred architecture is well documented (Mann 1993, Lawlor 1995) and it has a beneficial influence on the healing process, not least through the general sense of wellbeing that emerges in environments that make us feel at ease, inspire us and calm us. When people feel better through the presence of right relationship with their carer or the environment, they are more likely to get better (Kitson 1988). The proportions, entrances, layout and structure of buildings are believed to have a significant influence on those who use them. At one level, this refers to the pleasure such a building can give to the eye, the efficiency of the layout for working, the sights, sounds and smells it holds – all these can influence our sense of wellbeing in a place and affect our sense of connection with it; our right relationship with an environment is influenced by a much-loved building where we feel welcome and at home compared to one that feels impersonal and inhospitable. Thus, the notion is that if we get the healing environment right, get into right relationship with the environment in other words, the patients are far more likely to heal themselves.

Further studies have indicated the connection between buildings and wellness, varying from the aesthetics of the milieu, to proportions of buildings or the presence of geopathic stress (for example, Bachmann 1995, Soine 1995, von Pohl 1993, Freshwater 1997). There are growing signs of an increasing response to these issues, for example, the popularizing of Feng Shui, the Chinese art of balancing 'energies' in the environment (Rossbach 1992). Feng Shui is based on the Chinese concept of energy known as *ch'i*, and the expert practitioner seeks to generate a smooth flow of uninterrupted energy in the environment. This takes account of all manner of features: the shape of the building, the positioning of doors, mirrors, furniture, and so on. Freshwater (1997) notes that 'We are more than just a physical body, we are also that which we cannot see … as carers we cannot afford to ignore the dimensions that our senses cannot perceive'.

The concept of 'subtle energy' is still highly contentious, as we indicated in the Introduction. It may be a product of New Age imaginings or something real that, as yet, we do not have effective tools to measure. Thurnell-Read (1995), however, believes that 'We have an energy presence that can be disturbed by other energy presences, and we ignore this fact at our peril'. As yet, considerations of the energy of the environment have yet to be widely accepted in our healthcare systems. However, there are signs of change, as we have suggested, and as carers we have a significant part to play in exploring the relevance of both new and old knowledge in this field to our practice and in influencing the systems we work in to bring about change. As well as possibilities of intervention in building projects for the future, the present buildings, no matter how inappropriate to healthcare they can sometimes seem, are not beyond influence either.

Literature

Sacred words are often present in clinical areas. Indeed, few hotel rooms are without their Gideon's bible. At home or at work, it may be possible to provide more options.

The waiting room was full of the usual junk – ancient magazines, leftover newspapers, books that nobody wanted. We took a long, hard look at what was available and asked the patients what they would like to have available to read. With luck and good management, the waits were rarely long, so it was clear that people needed something that was concise and quickly read. Many people attending were often very sick and fearful. We produced leaflets about the major health problems that explained in simple language what was going on. We found books that contained inspiring words, or words to meditate or relax with. The Bible and the Qur'an were there, but we added all kinds of texts that we found in the bookshops, and invited patients to bring in works or tell us of books they could recommend. Some of it was poetry, great literature or short quotes from religious and spiritual texts. Sometimes these were profoundly significant to patients. I remember one old man being moved to tears and showing some words to me. 'This is just how I feel,' he said, 'this is just what it's like'. I used that to begin a dialogue with him that I feel really helped him to understand what was going on with him and how we could help. It broke the ice and, I think, it was a sort of healing for him to be able to talk for the first time about how he felt about his cancer rather than what he needed to know about the treatment and prospects. It made me take stock as well, about how blasé we can get with the endless passing through of patients, and how we can forget what a difficult place this is to be.

Texts that we have found useful in these type of instances include Ladouceur's (1996), Anderson's (1997) and Caddy's (1986) works, but there are many more available, and they all make a significant change from the dog-eared copies of weekly magazines that so often seem the only reading material on hand. For some people, a few pieces of innocuous literature are all that is wanted; others, however, may prefer something of greater significance, and it is important to ensure that an appropriate choice is available.

The hospital environment

Light, sound, smell and colour all help to shift our perceptions of the environment and affect our feelings of comfort or discomfort. This is easier to some degree in the private space of a person's home, where the individual's own choices can take precedence. It is rather more problematic in communal environments such as hospital wards where, for instance the burning of incense may inspire some patients but make others feel nauseous, as well as risking setting off a fire alarm! Such approaches therefore need to be used appropriately and with a good deal of caution. Margo Adair (cited in Biley 1996) writes how:

... we tend to forget our connection to the earth, to the sky, to each other, to the life that's constantly percolating in and around us. When we forget our connections, we wind up feeling drained and isolated. When we remember our connections, we become energised, inspired, and feel part of all that's around us.

I particularly remember Mrs Barlow. She had been incapacitated and speechless after a stroke, and I called in to see her before the round on Friday. She was, as usual, sat up in bed, with that same vacant stare on her face as the busy ward just flowed on around her. It was snowing hard, and for some reason, I just wanted her to see that there was still a big wide world out there. I told her, 'It's snowing, come and take a look, the fields and trees look lovely, and even the hospital buildings look pretty today'. I covered her with extra blankets, pushed her bed across to face the fire escape (the windows were too high for bedridden patients to see outdoors) and flung it open. The snow had stopped and the sky was clearing. Brilliant sunshine was shimmering in front of us. Some children had crossed from the park and were throwing snowballs and laughing hysterically at one another. I stepped out, made a snowball, and put it in her hand. She smiled a smile that I'd not seen in a long time, took the snowball to her forehead and wiped it across, then down across her lips then threw it at me! She lay there, enraptured, with a huge grin on her face.

Nightingale (1859) spoke eloquently of the need for light, fresh air, and pleasant sights and smells to raise the spirits and help towards a feeling of wellbeing. These old lessons are as applicable today as they were then, indeed as they were in the early Greek Aesculapian temples. Here, the temple-hospitals were 'built in places of great beauty so that patients could enjoy views, they were near natural springs so that the water could be pure and in raised positions so that there could be cooling breezes' (Biley 1996). Such an environment is a far cry from much of the world of the modern healthcare setting and people's homes. As we have suggested in the previous section, there is work to be done influencing the hospital plans for the future or taking advantage of the moment when plans for refurbishment are under way. Meanwhile, attention to the following can help to make a difference:

- Place bed and sitting areas where external views can be achieved.
- Select pictures that offer outdoor perspectives, such as landscapes, garden scenes and seascapes.
- Remember that patients who are bedridden may not be able to see walls or windows, so ceiling pictures and careful choice of ceiling illumination can be considered.
- Picture displays can be changed regularly.
- Develop collaborative relationships with artists to decorate clinical areas and corridors. Many such projects have been supported by arts councils and local and national charities (e.g. Arts for Health in Manchester).
- Rooms with windows are more likely to promote healing. In one US study (Biley 1996), it was found that patients without an outside view were likely to stay in hospital longer. Computerised false windows, to give the impression of clouds and the sun moving across the sky, have been used with success as a substitute.
- Well cared for plants not only help to clean the air and look and smell attractive, they can also be part of a therapeutic regime when patients are involved in caring for them. Large collections of plants can provide secluded areas in large open spaces and help to reduce noise.
- Colours used to decorate areas, or used to distinguish walkways or access areas can help to orientate patients. There is contention over choice of colours (the 'science' and 'art' of colour therapy for the home and office is now regularly advertised) and the impact upon staff and patients. Some colours and patterns appear to be more conducive to rest and sleep and certain mood states than others. Biley (1996) suggests that black and grey should be avoided, often being associated with death and struggle. Green and pink are often associated with healing, red with mood elevation, yellow with relieving depression, and so on. While the scientific evidence for the impact of colours is still somewhat tenuous, and there are enormous differences in cultural and personal preferences, there is no doubt that people perceive different impacts

in different coloured environments, and that colour is a factor to consider in making a place of healing more therapeutic.

- Noise is one of the most often cited causes of patient discomfort in hospitals and why the home is so much preferred. Some units have implemented quiet background music or gentle sounds of nature. Others have developed specific quiet periods during the day, when only minimal clinical activity is permitted.

> At 2 pm, we literally close the home. The doors are shut, and all potential visitors – GPs, district nurses, whoever – have been warned that this is a quiet hour. The staff may spend the time sitting quietly with patients, note writing, reading or in meditation. Some patients may use the time for prayer, others for sleep. Whatever the preference, everyone knows that this is the time of minimal activity during the day when we can all enjoy a few moments of calm and respite from the hurly burly of the usual daily activities.

> No matter what sort of busy day it's been, we all get together just for a few minutes to sit with Peter in peace and quiet. The whole family benefit from it, especially if Peter's had a difficult day. I may massage his legs or back, and he usually goes into a very calm state, almost like being in a trance. We darken the room, choose one of Peter's favourite bits of relaxing music, light a candle and burn some incense. The whole house is affected by it, and we all need this time when we can be together with a little peace.

Aldridge (1996) points to an extensive body of research indicating the positive benefits of music in the promotion of healing. From the relaxation effect of soft background music, to patient participation in music making, there are many opportunities for carers to find a path for music in holding the sacred in right relationship. Music, the 'food of love', has inspired people to the heights of human achievement, and has been used in all cultures as a meditative and contemplative tool to alter states of consciousness, from the repetitive drumming of the shaman to the ragas of India and the complex and intricate qawaal songs of the Sufis. Latterly, we have witnessed some of the most ground-breaking work in the care of the dying with the application of music at the point of death in the Chalice of Repose Project led by Dr Therese Schroeder-Sheker. A whole new (some might argue, renewed) science and art is emerging of 'music thanatology' (Schroeder-Sheker 1994): bringing prescriptive music to the dying and seriously ill with profound beneficial and spiritual effects being reported.

A full discussion of these and other topics related to environmental controls is beyond the scope of this text, but the examples cited above indicate that there is enormous potential for carers to use these techniques to create a healing, sacred context to benefit both themselves and those being cared for. On their own, these techniques may not be seen as particularly sacred: it is how we use them that seems to matter, and how they help us to shift our consciousness toward the sacred.

ALTARS AND SHRINES

Even the most drab of rooms, office, institution or home, can be transformed by creating a specific sacred space within it. A special corner, piece of furniture, window ledge – anywhere can be used to the same effect – a place of remembrance and reverence with objects that have meaning and significance for us. Peg Streep (1997) writes:

In our contemporary times, building altars – personal places of prayer, ritual and meditation – is one way of acknowledging the sacredness of all the space we inhabit, from the macrocosm of the blue planet to the microcosm of the home, the office and the garden. By acknowledging that something larger than ourselves with greater purpose exists, we create an environment where a sense of the sacred can be realised in the details of our everyday lives and in ourselves. Altars don't 'make' sacred space, they work by showing us what has been there all along.

I spend an enormous amount of time on the road, but no matter where I go, I always change my hotel room into my home. I've stayed in so many, they all begin to look the same after a while. A candle, my picture of Mother Meera, a crucifix, some flowers, some incense, a picture of my family – all these in one small spot can help me to feel more at ease, more present in that place (Plate 6). It is a focus for my attention when I pray or meditate. In fact, taking the trouble to make sure I pack these things and the preparation of the space itself becomes meditation.

According to the artist Meinrad Criaghead, the altar is 'the point where heaven and earth meet. The gods – spirits – come down and receive the offerings we place there to propitiate them. Any altar somehow partakes in the understanding of communion and of the power of the sacred objects that gather' (McCullogh 1997). Some religious bodies have grave misgivings about home-made altars, seeing them as places of 'heathen' worship. However, it is important to distinguish between worship and reverence. The objects on the altar are not for worship as things in themselves; rather, they are present to focus our attention, our consciousness, upon the sacred though the medium of things which have special meaning for us. The very act of creating the altar seems to make us more spiritually receptive, more open to the sacred, as well as providing us with a focus for our own spiritual practice. It is the connection that seems to make a place sacred, the bringing of the artefacts, the setting up, the concentration and the effort involved, and not just the objects in themselves.

My office has become my own sacred space. Laid out all around are objects that have importance and significance for me in my spiritual life, which is also my daily life. There is no difference to me. The cross upon the wall, my Buddha in the window alcove, the flowers and crystals I have placed there, all these things and more have made my place of work a place of special significance to me. My colleagues at first were very wary, and some I know thought I was completely crackers. But I notice that others have started to do likewise. It's interesting to see how my little space has become the one where everyone gravitates to eventually – 'yours is the only place that seems calm here', 'it's a haven of peace' – these are the sort of things they say. People prefer to meet here, they say the meetings are always so much more productive. It may of course just be me that they come to, that creates that kind of atmosphere, but there's more to it than that, in my view. Just creating a beautiful space has an effect on people, especially one that would otherwise be just another office like all the rest of the rooms in this very boring building. It's interesting, too, how colleagues have added to the space over the years. My own sacred space has accumulated gifts – feathers, stones, crystals – gathered by my fellow workers while on holidays or trips away. I love the idea that they should think of this space and how to contribute to it, even though they might be far away.

Altars can be created at home or at work. They can become places where carers and cared for can place objects of special reverence to them. They can be simple affairs or more complex ones. At Commonweal in the USA, an important centre for cancer care and social change, clients may spend time communally constructing an altar during their stay. We have visited hospital wards where a simple icon or crucifix is placed at patients' bedsides at their request; other places where intricate arrangements have been built up several feet high. From an icon in the corner of an office to a pergola in a garden, the options for constructing an altar are many and varied. Murray (1997) describes most beautifully how a part, or indeed the whole, of our garden can become a place of reverence. Arrangements of plants, furniture, walls or sculpture can create the same effect outdoors as in. All generations and all cultures have sought to make gardens sacred places of reverence, prayer, meditation and contemplation. Murray points out that 'Our gardens can provide a a place of deep connection and belonging, where we can express our personal identities and form relationships with our space, our plants, ourselves'. And it may be, as we cultivate or spend time in the beauty of a garden, that synchronicity enters our lives – beauties begin to enter our lives in other arenas to match the beauty we contemplate in the sacred space of the garden. Recognising this healing power of the garden, more and more health institutions have paid attention to the maintenance of both outdoor gardens and indoor plants. Even a small piece of ground or part of a room can become a natural altar of peace and harmony to nourish the soul.

On a recent visit to Washington for Memorial Day, we were moved to see the thousands of visitors to the great black marble wall dedicated to those who died in Vietnam. With its flowers, icons and other mementos, this great space had become a giant altar, a shrine to loss, suffering and remembrance. Not far away, however, we witnessed the creation of another sacred space. This time, there was more a sense of gratitude as well as loss. Thousands of men and women crossed the park to lay poems, flowers, cards of praise and thanks, and prayers at the feet of a simple group of life-size bronze statues dedicated to the nurses who served in the conflict. People stood in silence, exchanged reminiscences, wept – all around these simple figures (Plate 7). Amid the death and destruction of war, the acts of terror and of heroism, something else had been noticed that was worthy of remembrance: the acts of love and compassion. A simple collection of statues had become an altar to some of the finest acts of human behaviour, the capacity of some who care to 'Keep their hearts open in hell' (Ram Dass & Bush 1992).

Nowadays, the need in people to express connection with an event at a particular place seems greater than ever, whether it be to commemorate a loss or something of joy. It seems that no roadside is free of its pile of flowers where an accident has taken place. Parts of the city of London were buried in flowers following the death of Princess Diana in 1997. We find and create places where we can express our feelings as both individuals and communities, dedicating them in thanksgiving or sorrow. Sacred space can be found in every corner of our lives, if we choose to seek it out.

LABYRINTHS

A labyrinth is a path or walkway built on sacred geometric principles, which we enter, walk a specified, meandering route and return to the same point that we started on. Of the spiritual journey, T S Eliot (1943) writes in the *Four Quartets*:

> We shall not cease from exploration
> And the end of all our exploring
> Will be to arrive where we started
> and know the place for the first time.

Walking a labyrinth can have that same quality to it as we deepen insights into ourselves. Artress (1995) sees labyrinths as 'divine imprints ... they are universal patterns most likely created in the collective unconscious, birthed through the human psyche and passed down through the ages. Labyrinths are mysterious because we do not know the origin of their design, or exactly how they provide space that allows clarity'. A labyrinth is a not a maze, with its blind alleys and traps. There is only one way in and one way out and, as it twists and turns, we are guided through all points of the compass and phases of the moon until we reach the centre. The path may mirror our path through life, sometimes seeming lost, sometimes seeming to go backwards, but always the point ahead remains the same.

Labyrinths have been used throughout human history in many designs, the simplest being the universal spiral shape, regularly found depicted on the neolithic tombs of Western Europe (Fig. 4.3).

This archetypal shape, with its spiritual significance, is found in many variations at some stage in all cultures. Indeed, all labyrinths, however complex their layout may seem to be, are based on the same essential spiral shape. The spiral can be seen as our path through life as we move out into the world from the centre; likewise it mirrors our return from the world to

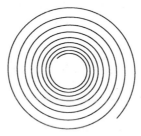

Figure 4.3   The universal spiral shape.

our source. 'The circular path inward cleanses and quiets as it leads us in. The unwinding path integrates and empowers us on our walk back out. Walking out of the winding path we are literally ushered back out into the world in a strengthened condition' (Artress 1995).

With a little imagination, it is possible to walk a labyrinthine route around the streets near our homes or places of work. As with so many of the techniques discussed in this chapter, a large part of the impact is determined by our preparation, commitment and actions as we follow a particular path. The process is as important as the outcome. Many people, when troubled, facing a difficult decision or unable to solve a problem, instinctively take a walk. This purposeful walking is clearly related to the principle of walking the labyrinth. The latter, however, with its sacred geometric principles, is thought to be a more powerful tool to work with. It is possible to create a simple labyrinth in the home or garden or at work: all that is needed is a space about 4 m across. Mark out a cross in the centre, and mark four points, for example, with stones or cardboard pieces (Figure 4.4A) then join the dots (Figure 4.4B–E)

For further information on labyrinth construction, especially the precise geometric proportions (which are very important as the first section on sacred geometry indicated) we strongly recommend the reader to turn to texts by

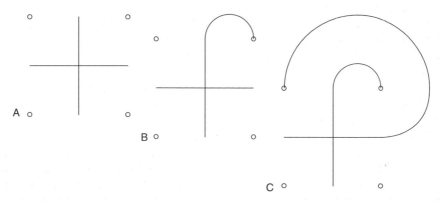

Figure 4.4

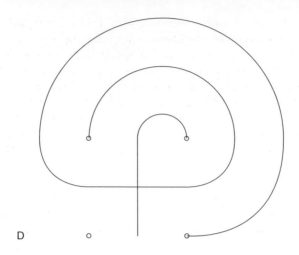

D

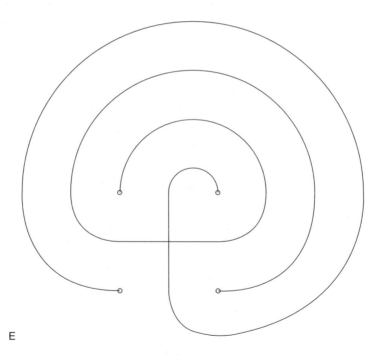

E

Figure 4.4 *Cont'd* Creating a simple labyrinth. (A) Stage 1 (B) Stage 2 (C) Stage 3 (D) Stage 4 (E) Stage 5.

Sig Lonegrin (1991) and Lauren Artress (1995). Like all the paths discussed in this chapter, none of them should be undertaken lightly.

There are many possible labyrinth designs, and the one we have shown here is one of the simplest and easiest to create. More complex ones have been designed throughout human history, probably reaching a zenith with the labyrinth in Chartres Cathedral. Lying almost unknown and unused for several hundred years after its construction in the 12th century, the Chartres Labyrinth was given a new lease of life after its 'rediscovery' and more widespread dissemination through the work of Dr Lauren Artress, Canon for Special Ministries at Grace Cathedral in San Francisco (Plate 8), and her colleagues in the Veriditas Project. Since then, there has been an increasing uptake in the use of labyrinths of the Chartres design formed from 11 concentric circles with a 12th being the centre of the labyrinth (Figure 4.5). The path meanders throughout the whole circle. The centre has six petals or rosettes; the rose and its eastern equivalent, the lotus, are almost universally regarded as symbols of enlightenment, even today. The labyrinth has a feminine quality to it, emphasised in the labyrs or double-axe symbols visible at the turns; the double-axe is traditionally seen as a symbol of women's power and creativity. The feminine quality continues with the

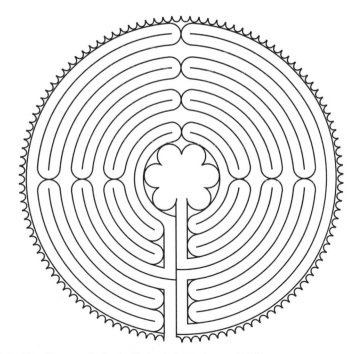

Figure 4.5   The Chartres Cathedral Labyrinth (Anderson 1992).

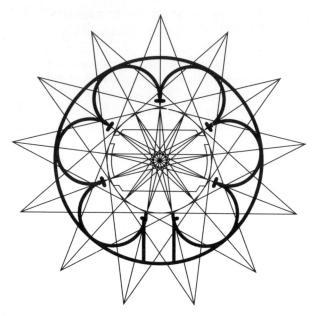

Figure 4.6   The 13-point star at the centre of the Chartres Labyrinth (Anderson 1992)

lunations, which consist of 28 points per quadrant. In addition, the precise geometric proportions form an invisible 13 pointed star that radiates from its centre, one of the most important and significant features of the labyrinth form. This invisible star seems to 'empower the labyrinth in some inexplicable way' (Artress 1995).

Portable labyrinths can be made, and the authors have one which we have taken to local churches, conferences and so on (Plate 9). A wooden design, small enough to be held in the hand, is also available. This can be used by placing a finger in the groove marking the route and following it to the centre as a quiet meditative practice. It allows us, therefore, to have convenient access to the qualities of the labyrinth wherever we wish. It is especially useful when we cannot access a full-scale version, or for those who have difficulty walking. The effects that people report are the same as those documented by Artress (1995): for example, problems being solved, profound insights into the self, feeling guided by the divine.

When the labyrinth was laid out in the churchyard, it looked beautiful under the summer sun. It seemed to draw you into walking. I felt this most strongly, and me a diehard skeptic. I remember thinking cynically, 'Look at all these silly people here, they're fantasising, you won't get me making a spectacle of myself like that' … I don't know to this day how I ended up walking it. The next thing I remember, I was stood at the entrance, many others were ahead of me. I remember the brilliant blue of the sky, I looked up at the sun, uttered a brief prayer and walked.

I remember irritation as people passed me, or I had to stop and let others by, I remember feeling angered by people ahead of me who seemed so slow. I remember feeling lost, that I was never going to get out of it, of seeming close to the centre, only to be thrown back to walk another arc that took me away from it. At the centre, I stopped, prayed again, sat for a while. I suddenly felt incredibly clean, like I had just taken a cool shower. I looked around and saw how everyone was moving at their own pace, fast or slow, stumbling or purposeful, turning, passing, going back and coming forward, and I just felt so blissful, at ease like I could barely remember before ... and such love and appreciation for all those like me who were just making their journey. We were all the same, great or small, black or white, old or young, in the end I realised we are all the same, everyone is just doing this. This is life.

When walking a spiral or labyrinth, it is necessary to follow a few simple rules (based on Artress 1995):

• Before entering, spend a few moments in reflection on where you are in your life. You may find a focus, a question, statement or prayer that you may wish to take in with you.

• Do not enter with any expectation of results; this sets you up for disappointment. Go in with an open heart and mind.

• Move through the labyrinth at a pace, time and manner that feel right to you, but remember to have respect for others who may be in there with you, especially if you wish to move past or around them.

• On entering you can try:

— gracious attention: quiet the mind, let all thoughts go, just allow a sense of calmness yet wakefulness to flow through you

— asking a question: focusing on a question that you have been asking yourself, outside the realm of yes and no answers; be open to whatever comes in; do not try to control or create expectations of a particular answer

— use of repetition: using a mantra or other word or phrase which you repeat. It could be one that has meaning for you, or one that is meaningless, simply serving to quiet the mind and keep yourself open to whatever comes in

— reading scripture: words that inspire you or feel right for you, from your own faith or other books on spirituality, or poetry or general literature

— asking for help through prayer: by praying throughout the walk.

Other ways to use a spiral or labyrinth might be:

• honouring a benchmark in time such as a birthday or special festival
• using bodily movement as prayer and meditation
• letting your ego go, the impatient judgemental thoughts that keep us from hearing the still, small place within
• bringing a dream with you that you want to remember or make clear
• just experiencing whatever comes to you.

Afterwards you might want to write about your experience or express it in some other way such as drawing, painting or sharing it with a friend. Be cautious in how you interpret what happens. It is often difficult to differentiate between imagination and revelation. Consider what happens as guidance for thought and action, for work and interpretation, rather than as fixed results.

Labyrinths have begun to be reintroduced in churches, gardens, public parks, and in hospitals, where both staff and patients have made use of them. The authors are involved in several such projects at the moment, one to restore a long-neglected one in a local college, another to construct one in a busy town centre, and another in the grounds of a hospital as part of a 'caring for the carers' project.

Labyrinths appear to be helpful in many ways, ranging from a simple relaxation effect to divine inspiration. Much more research is needed, and the Veriditas project has already accumulated a considerable body of evidence, mostly individual narratives. Labyrinths warrant serious consideration for reintegration into our everyday lives, as tools for the sacred, and as helpmates on our spiritual journey.

MEDITATION

Hebrew scriptures tell the story of the prophet Elijah. Hiding in a cave, in fear for his life, he waited for God. An earthquake followed, almost sending the cave crashing down upon him. Still he did not hear or see God. Then a great fire came rushing by, and still he did not hear or see God, even in this awesome display of power. Afterwards, a deep silence settled upon the cave, silence so profound that it spoke. In silence, the voice he sought was heard.

Meditation is a method by which a person empties the mind of all thoughts, stimuli and expectations while, paradoxically, becoming more alert. Christine Longaker (1998) suggests that:

Instead of looking outward toward the world, in meditation we shift our attention inward, to help us connect with our innermost essence – a pure, boundless awareness and natural simplicity. Training in meditation, we can experience breaks in our endless mental suffering – moments of freedom, spaciousness and deep peace (Figure 4.6). By committing ourselves to study, contemplation, and meditation, we can learn to sustain and integrate into our entire way of being the openness, clarity and boundless compassion of our true nature, until we transcend suffering entirely.

Thus meditation, by centring ourselves, helps us to be easier in the world and thereby more available to others with that 'boundless compassion'. Likewise, people who are ill have reported a wide range of benefits from meditation, finding themselves better placed for healing to occur.

The meditation group at the hospital had small beginnings. At first, it grew from just three of us who, by chance, discovered that we were all meditators, although we all used different methods. Eventually, after a teacher came in and did a series of introductory classes, the group increased to around 20 regulars. Apart from helping us as individuals, we believe there is an add-on effect in our homes and places of work. We all work in fairly frantic units, but if we can remain calm and centred most of the time, then that can influence our colleagues and our patients, if there's one less person falling apart in this place, then it helps to take some of the madness out it. It gets reduced, if only by one less person, but perhaps by others who are affected by being near us. Now we try to ensure that at least one of us has meditated on the wellbeing of the workplace each day. Our goal is that, at every point during the day, at least one person is always in meditation in the hospital. There have been many claims, for example by those in the TM [transcendental meditation] movement that crime, stress, violence and so on in a community can be reduced if only a small percentage meditate. The meditators can influence all around them in many subtle ways. We are intrigued to see if that might happen here.

Meditation tends to focus on personal and experiential rather than intellectual knowledge – a deepening of understanding of ourselves and our relationship with the beyond. It shifts our attention from active, outward consciousness and events, to what is taking place inside us. Meditation is essentially a practice discipline and needs to be experienced to learn it. What follows is a summary of a number of key points as a guide to understanding the nature and purpose of meditation. Any reader who wishes to understand meditation in depth and to practice it would be well advised to find a suitable source for teaching and support. Learning to meditate may take hard work and discipline, and it is a process through which we never stop learning. Likening the inner world to an 'interior castle', St Teresa of Avila (1995) wrote 'As far as I can understand, the gate by which to enter this castle is prayer and meditation'.

Much of the teaching of meditation in Europe has been greatly influence by eastern philosophy and approaches in recent years. Indeed, Carl Jung is said to have believed that the greatest impact upon western thinking at the end of the millennium will come from the integration of Buddhist psychology (Storr 1996). And yet western European traditions also include methods akin to eastern practices, such as contemplation within the Christian tradition. Whatever the source, meditation techniques appear to have a number of features in common, and Larry LeShan's (1974) text still provides one of the best introductions to the theme that we can recommend.

First, there is much evidence to indicate that meditation produces a state of physical and mental relaxation, promoting a sense of wellbeing, reducing stress and anxiety, improving the autoimmune response and helping with the healing of damaged tissue. On this basis, nurses and other healthcare workers who experience stressful occupations might benefit from it, as may their patients. Second, it can induce a state of calm in which we can think through difficulties, solve problems and set them in context, deepen our understanding and gain insight into ourselves. Third, meditation can help us to be 'fully human' (LeShan 1974), to expand our consciousness and go beyond insight into life's daily difficulties and the need to relax into a deeper awareness of who we are, how to be in the world and our relationship with our innermost self, and perhaps our God.

Contemplation can be seen as focusing with our eyes or with our mind upon a particular object or thought (for example, the Christian contemplative who looks upon the cross to gain insight or union with God), or simply concentrating upon a particular word, idea or inspiring object, such as a flower. Meditation usually refers to inwardly coming to a place of calm and absence of judgemental thought. The two approaches are closely related but quite distinct, although they have often been used interchangeably. An enormous variety of techniques is available. Every culture and every spiritual discipline has developed meditative and contemplative techniques of one form or another throughout history. Indeed, one of the problems for the beginner is finding the right one for him- or herself. LeShan (1995) comments on meditation: 'To me there is no one right way. What's right for one person is wrong for another. There's no one right diet for cancer for example. I've seen people do beautifully on the macrobiotic diet and I've seen people damn near die of it – not of the disease, but of the diet. There's no one right way'. Some practitioners have sought to merge techniques with good effect, for example, MacInnes' (1996) work with Buddhist and Christian approaches.

Many traditions, such as the Quakers (Religious Society of Friends) use sitting in silence to worship and connect with the 'voice within'. The notion of listening to the inner voice in silence, perhaps receiving divine guidance, is a common approach in the west. Work such as that of Eileen Caddy (1971) follows this trend, echoing the revelatory nature which comes from a place of inner stillness, going far back into European history, for example, in the writings of Julian of Norwich, Hildegard of Bingen or St Teresa of Avila. The idea of just 'sitting' – being physically and mentally still – and allowing the mind to become quiet and detach from the stimuli of the everyday world (Kamalashila 1988), underpins many meditative and contemplative techniques.

Other traditions, such as Buddhism, seek to come to a point of stillness in meditation where there is a complete absence of thought or sensation, simply dwelling in a state of open awareness and being absolutely present 'in the moment'. This state is known as 'sky of mind' or 'diamond consciousness'. A further aim is to bring this state of consciousness into everyday reality: just being present with full attention in every moment. This contrasts with meditation techniques which some schools of thought would not see as meditation in which the meditator seeks to solve problems or to go on some inner journey to seek help or new insights and awareness. Such an altered state of consciousness occurs in shamanic techniques, can be induced by drugs, or similar effects can be attained using guided meditation. In the latter, the meditator is asked to visualize a particular scene or follow a particular sequence of events to seek insights. For example:

Sit quietly and comfortably with your eyes closed in a quiet and darkened room. Bring your attention to your breathing and relax as you follow the rise and fall of your breath. Imagine yourself on a warm summer's day, sitting by a clear pool completely alone. The grass is green, a gentle breeze wafts the trees and the sky is radiant blue in bright sunshine.

Just sit and enjoy this pleasant scene for a moment, and after a little while, you begin to notice that there is something else present. You sense that a creature is nearby ... it may be a bird of the air, an animal on land or something in the water. You turn to face it, and notice its warmth and friendliness towards you. It approaches and you sense that it has something to say to you. It may speak, or whisper, or mouth the words, or may move or gesture in a particular way. You sense that there is a special message just for you, and you take note of it and keep it in the back of your mind or hold it close in your heart. You may spend a little more time with your creature, but then it is time to say goodbye. You give thanks for whatever message you have been given, and knowing now that this is a special place that belongs only to you, and to which you can return at any time, you slowly allow yourself to open your eyes and become aware of the room.

Such 'visualising' types of meditation contrast with the emptying of thought and sensation that are part of the Buddhist tradition (Figure 4.7). Other techniques may involve movement and/or music and rhythm. The

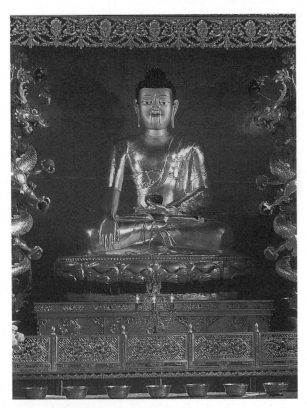

Figure 4.7 Buddhism has had a profound influence on our understanding of meditation. © Forder & Forder, reprinted with permission.

mystical path of the Sufis follows a passion for music and dance as their meditation, expressed in this poem by Rumi (quoted in Harvey 1994):

How could the soul not take flight
When from the glorious presence
A soft call flows sweet as honey, comes right up to her
and whispers, 'Rise up now, come away.'
How could the fish not jump
Immediately from dry land into water
When the sound of water from the ocean
Of fresh waves springs to his ear?
How could the hawk not fly away
Forgetful of all hunting to the wrist of the king
As soon as he hears the drum
The king's baton hits again and again,
Drumming out the signal of return?
How could the Sufi not start to dance,
Turning on himself, like the atom, in the sun of eternity,
So he can leap free of this dying world?
Fly away, fly away bird to your native home,
You have leapt free of the cage
Your wings are flung back in the wind of God.
Leave behind the stagnant and marshy waters,
Hurry, hurry, hurry, o bird, to the source of life!

Harvey also writes of the spiritual practice of some Sufis, known to some of the outside world as 'whirling dervishes'.

The dervishes, with arms crossed and hands on each other's shoulders, begin to dance slowly. They extend their arms like wings, the right hand turned up toward heaven to receive the divine grace, the left hand turned toward the earth to direct the divine grace that is coming into the right hand down onto the earth. Circling, they dance around the room. This dance around the room symbolizes union in plurality: the dancers unite themselves with everything in the cosmos that is also dancing (union in plurality), but it is also the whole dance of existence, the dance of evolution through all its stages of ascension, from stone to man.

To whirl like a dervish might not be appealing for everyone. Meditations can also be developed around everyday activities such as eating. Indeed, many people can experience a meditative-like state simply by becoming very focused on a particular task, such as concentrating on a hobby, painting, writing, sports activities and so on. Many Buddhist schools teach that being fully present in the moment, with whatever that moment holds, is the purpose of meditation.

Some techniques focus on bodily rhythms to achieve a meditative state. For example:

Sit quietly with your eyes closed in a quiet room. Begin to count your breathing. Count each time you exhale up to a count of four, then inhale and count again from one to four. Continue to do this so that you become aware only of your breathing and your counting. See how long you can keep this up before you lose count or your mind begins to wander.

Such techniques help to calm the mind and relax us, and they can also show how tense and anxious we are, how easily the mind wanders, and how difficult it is to stay focused on a task as simple as counting our breath. One of the goals of meditation is, through practice, to develop the skill and attention that help us to master the will and the mind that distract us, and to bring that degree of focused, quiet attention into our daily lives.

To help induce a relaxed state or alter our consciousness so that we become more open, aware and focused in our meditation, many aids have been developed. These include:

• Particular postures or movements, such as the classic 'lotus' position (sitting cross legged, with feet over both thighs), the many positions known in yoga techniques, or the movements associated with T'ai chi and chi qung.

• Smell: the use of incense for example.

• Sound: adding suitable background music, or the use of chants and mantras (words or phrases repeated verbally or silently in the mind to induce a state of quietness and attention. These may be well-established words, such as the great 'aum' or 'om', they may given by a teacher, be taken from inspiring books, or we may make up our own).

• Focusing on bodily rhythms, e.g. breathing.

• Visual techniques, for example, the use of an inspiring picture, icon, view, flowers and so on, or the use of special lighting such as a candle in a shaded room.

• Meditative pathways, for example, labyrinths such as that in Chartres Cathedral.

These and other techniques are often used in various forms and combinations to induce a meditative state. However, it is necessary to be cautious about getting caught up in materialism around spiritual matters; 'I can't meditate because I haven't got my favourite crystal/music/charm or whatever with me'. It is important to see these as tools to help towards a meditative state rather than ends in themselves. It is also necessary to be careful how we interpret the information that we sometimes receive in meditation, as the mind can play many tricks on us (see Chapter 5).

Some further general guidance for meditation that we suggest is:

• If using a sitting meditation, choose a posture that is most comfortable for you. Particular schools use particular methods, but a comfortable chair offering an upright position may be all that you need. Avoid lying down if you want to avoid falling sleep.

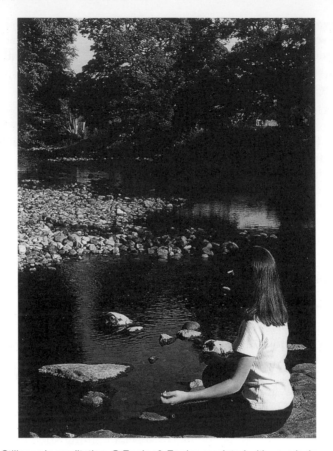

Figure 4.8 Stillness in meditation. © Forder & Forder, reprinted with permission.

- Prepare your environment, especially prepare a special sacred place and time if this is possible. Experienced meditators may say that they can meditate anywhere, but for the novice it is usually necessary to have:
  — a quiet, undisturbed room
  — lighting adjusted to a comfortable level
  — even, comfortable temperature
  — a cushion or suitable chair for comfort, perhaps with a blanket or shawl to cover the body
  — music, incense, candles or other aids according to your choice or method
  — removed interruptions, e.g. the telephone or telling others not to disturb you
- Read and study widely about the options for meditation, find a technique that suits you and pursue it in depth.

- Find a good teacher and/or course and/or group of like-minded others where you can be given expert tuition, guidance and support. But, be very wary of 'gurus' who ask you to surrender yourself, your body or your money to them in return for their 'unique' knowledge! Meditation is an empowering process for you, it does not ask you to surrender yourself to others. (See Chapter 5 for more on this theme.)

- Relax into your meditation technique – whatever is happening is meant to be happening. Avoid getting too outcome-orientated, and avoid trying to judge your meditations as good or bad. If you fall asleep, that's all right, it's what you needed. If it seemed confused, that's all right too. What did it teach you about your state of mind? You can always come back to it later.

- Develop a routine. Part of your own sacred space might be to allocate a specific time each day when you will meditate, and then commit yourself to it as far as possible. Perhaps an hour each morning or evening, or whatever feels right for you. Even five minutes each day can be beneficial. Make sure others know that this is your time for yourself, and that you cannot be interrupted. If using meditation in the work situation, establish a pattern so that everyone is aware that a certain time is dedicated to contemplation, prayer or meditation, as given in the example in the previous section of this chapter.

- Keep a reflective diary or journal of your experiences, which you can share with trusted colleagues or your teacher, and use as a reference point to observe how your practice is developing.

There is a story of a Buddhist master who was teaching a meditation class to a group of westerners. One excitedly said to the master that he had a wonderful meditation – 'It was filled with light and bliss, and I felt like I was in heaven'. Another, trying to outdo the first, told of his meeting with the Divine, of flashing blue lights, and yet another, not to be outdone, told of her meeting with her dead grandmother and many other 'spirits'. 'Never mind,' the master said to his students, 'maybe tomorrow your meditations will be better!'. We need to be cautious about only seeking the blissful meditative experience, as this too can become a trap that keeps us from moving on and deepening our practice.

Eventually, it is possible to reach a stage where many of the accoutrements of meditation are unnecessary, and we lose any dependence upon outside circumstances. As we develop our practice, meditation is integrated into our whole way of being, and the occasions when we can be said to be 'in meditation' differ little from our everyday lives. No matter where we are, in a busy street or completing some household chore, in a frantic airport or in the centre of a city – the quietness and stillness we need for meditation, the sacred place, are always with us. We come to carry it around inside ourselves.

In this brief introduction to meditation, it has been possible only to skim the surface of a few of its many facets. Many meditation techniques are available, and it is important for each person to select a method that is right for them. Because of its generally beneficial effects upon the practitioner, it would seem to be a suitable practice for healthcare workers and lay carers to bring into our lives, and to introduce to those we care for. Indeed, many healthcare settings are making meditation part of the daily routine or prescribing it for patients with certain stress-related health problems.

Meditation can help us to find meaning and purpose in a world which is often confusing and perplexing. Many teachers of meditation believe that the benefits reach out beyond the individual. If we are more relaxed and attentive in our lives, then that impacts upon others around us. They too can feel more calm in the presence of someone who seems centred and unruffled. With practice, it can deepen our understanding of ourselves and our place in the grander scheme of things. We become easier in the world and better able to relax into the 'all that is'. In doing so, we may receive revelation and inspiration that to some is divine in origin. We may find ourselves relaxing into the possibility that not just ourselves, but the whole universe, is in a state of meditation. There is an intriguing phrase from the Upanishads which says:

Meditation, assuredly is more than thought. The earth meditates, as it were. The atmosphere meditates, as it were. Heaven meditates, as it were. Gods and men meditate, as it were. Hence those among men here who attain greatness – they are as it were, a part of the estate of meditation. Now, those who are small are quarrelers, malingerers, slanderers. But those who are superior – they are, as it were, a part of the estate of meditation. Therefore value meditation. (Easwaran 1988)

Meditation is therefore:

... playful, creative, alertness, your nature, non-doing, witnessing, a jump, scientific, an experiment, silence, paradise, remembrance, freedom, sensitivity, growing up, not escapist, clarity, emptiness, intelligence, cleansing, a flowering, awareness, fun, understanding, delight, relaxation, cool, oneness, recreation, rest, mastery, in the gap, in the present, a happening, transformation, coming home, living joyously. (Osho 1995)

In short, meditation is an adventure for the body, heart, mind and soul.

PRAYER

Religious commitment has been shown in a wide range of studies to be related to better health, although it seems, as Benson (1996) and Ornish (1998) report, that it is not just religious faith that is likely to keep us well, but any sense of connection to others in a community or group, be it a religious order or a football team. Herbert Benson's (1996) review of the extensive body of available research indicates that:

The greater a person's commitment, the fewer his or her psychological problems, the better his or her general health, the lower the blood pressure, the longer the survival. Across the board, in groups of different ages, ethnicites and religions, among patients with very different diseases and conditions, religious commitment brings with it a lifetime of benefits.

Yet, as the Rev. David Stoter (1995) suggests, the impact of a person's religion is largely ignored by healthcare professionals. It seems that, in an attempt to be studiously non-judgemental or to avoid seeming preferential, the role of providing religious support has been almost exclusively handed over to others, such as hospital chaplains. Carers themselves report how difficult it is to talk about their religious beliefs at work; not that they wish to convert others to their point of view, but they wish to have views shared as a normal topic of conversation and discuss how they might integrate their own practices with patients' requests and needs.

As a practising Christian, my faith has been a tower of strength to me in meeting all the pain and suffering that I encounter with patients every day. I don't ask people to believe what I believe, or to do as I do, but I do find that there is great difficulty among my healthcare colleagues in even seeing a need, let alone asking for help for patients. Patients themselves seem diffident about mentioning their faith to doctors and nurses; the staff, if they ask at all, seem to do no more than find the religious 'label' but then do not pursue inquiries to see if the patient has any special needs – such as an opportunity to be quiet and prayerful, a space on the ward where they can have a moment's peace and so on. If somewhere like Manchester airport can provide multi-faith prayer room for all passengers, then surely our hospitals and nursing homes can too?

I'm also saddened to see how difficult it is to talk about faith generally, it seems to have become a taboo subject. I went to see one of my patients in hospital, which as it happens has a good chaplaincy service, but she was uncomfortable about asking for more. I knew her well, as a member of my own church, so I did not hesitate to spend a few moments in prayer with her, and then ask the staff on her behalf to ensure that she could see the chaplain, receive communion and have time in her daily schedule set aside to be alone. It's not that the service was unavailable, or that the staff did not care. It seems that patients don't like to trouble the staff with 'I believe in God, and while here I would appreciate this, this or this'. And staff in general are just too plain embarrassed or ignorant to know how to respond if a patient did.

It seems that it is still very difficult for carers to take account of a person's religious beliefs in day-to-day care. Many healthcare settings do provide on-site chapels and chaplaincy services and, in a multicultural society, attempt to make these multi-faith as well. In institutions, there are signs of a growing recognition of the need to educate staff in the needs of patients from different religious backgrounds. More and more organisations are ensuring that a chaplain is available to the sick 24 hours a day, and are encouraged in the UK, by policy developments along these lines in the National Health Service (Dix 1996). At a more personal level, however, staff involved in caring often find it much more difficult to help patients with prayer, especially in participating themselves.

Mrs Gibbs had only been in the [nursing] home for two weeks, but it looked like this was going to be her home for the rest of her life. As the realisation dawned on her, she was obviously very troubled. I spent some time with her, as I would with any resident, just giving her time to talk about how she felt. I was shocked when she turned to me and said, 'it would help if you would just pray with me, nurse'. I was taken aback. On reflection, a patient had never asked me to do this in eight years of nursing. No one in nursing school had taught us how to respond to this one. And I hadn't been in a church for donkey's years. I told her this, but she said it didn't matter, she asked me just to sit with her and close my eyes, and she said a few words asking for God's help and guidance and things like that. It felt right to do this, just sit with her in silence as she spoke. In fact, I felt like it was me who was being nursed. The patient had taken charge and was telling me what to do.

Although I still do not have very strong beliefs myself, that incident made me much more aware of the gaps in my care for others. It is interesting here at the hospice – the approach is very different. To pray with patients at their request is seen as ordinary as meeting their toilet needs. No one gives it a second thought, and we set aside a quiet time just after breakfast when the whole place becomes still for a little while, prayers are said, out in the main patient area for those who are not mobile, and in the chapel. I was skeptical about this at first, wondering how patients who do not have strong beliefs might respond, but I was surprised to find that it is something that everyone appreciates, even non-believers.

The difference between prayer and meditation is not always clear, but a simple approach might be 'prayer is when I talk to God; meditation is when I listen.' If meditation is about stilling the mind, prayer involves active request and thinking. Helping with prayer may be something that professional carers have not been generally taught, and it may be more difficult for us when we are asked to participate. Yet prayer has been demonstrated to have a direct impact on people's wellbeing (Benson 1996, Dossey 1996) (Figure 4.9). People who are prayed for are more likely to get well compared to those who are not, and it seems to make little difference what denominational background they are from, or whether or not they know that they are being prayed for (Dossey 1996). This opens up a whole new and fascinating field in the study of human consciousness, and the possibilities of intercessionary prayer and other forms of 'wellwishing' for others.

Professional carers have always been taught to obtain a person's consent before any intervention. At the same time, some activities seem so fundamental that consent seems not to be an issue, such as providing food and shelter, rescuing someone in harm's way, or helping the sick and dying. Does prayer also fall into this category? Dossey (1996), in an excellent study on prayer, writes that 'some of us don't give much thought to consent issues when we pray because we suspect prayer may not work in the first place. If prayer is ineffective, consent doesn't matter. But what if prayer is more effective than we think?' Some see prayer as an invasion of privacy. Some see it as an invasion of their souls. One can see how intrusive prayer might seem to some, for instance if you were being prayed for (as Dossey reports) by someone who took the advice of an American evangelist who suggested on television: 'You

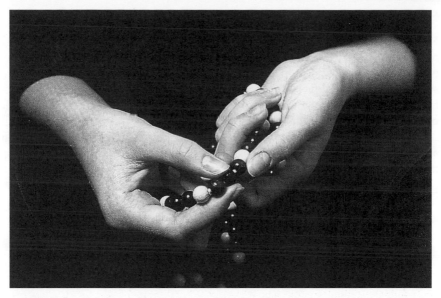

Figure 4.9   Prayer has a direct impact on wellbeing. © Forder & Forder, reprinted with permission.

can actually tell God what you would like his part in the covenant to be!' Complicating this issue is considerable evidence that prayer can harm as well as heal: 'Several scientific experiments show that we can retard biological processes in living organisms as well as help or stimulate them, at a distance, without the awareness of the recipient. This implies that prayer, like any drug or surgical procedure, has potential side effects' (Dossey 1996).

However, there is a form of prayer that avoids most of the problems of consent, privacy and invasion, in which we simply pray 'Thy will be done'. With this kind of prayer we are neither inflicting our personal wishes on another, nor playing the role that is God's.

Dossey reports a quote from Gandhi:

Prayer has saved my life ... I had my share of the bitterest public and private experiences. They threw me into temporary despair. If I was able to get rid of that despair it was because of prayer ... It came out of sheer necessity as I found myself in a plight where I could not possibly be happy without it. And as time went on, my faith in God increased and more irresistible became the yearning for prayer. Life seemed to be dull and vacant without it ... In spite of despair staring me in the face on the political horizon, I have never lost my peace ... That peace comes from prayer ... I am indifferent as to the form. Everyone is a law unto himself in that respect ... Let everyone try and find that as a result of daily prayer he adds something new to his life.

Dossey ends his book, '... in the spirit of tolerance and simplicity ... may you embark on your individual journey of prayer ... a solitary journey, but it need not be lonely. Why should it be? ... if you pray for me, and I for you...'.

SANCTUARY

Preparing ourselves to work compassionately in the world, in right relationship, may mean that for many of us, a time away from our usual everyday activities is helpful. Many organizations offer 'retreat' facilities, some allied to a specific religious or belief system, others with specific courses in mind of a more generic nature. At the Sacred Space Foundation, for example, professional carers can spend time in seclusion, resting quietly and meditating alone, working with a teacher, or joining in groupwork to learn about healing techniques, right relationship or meditation. Many of the great mystics, meditation teachers and therapists cited in this text give examples of the need to step aside from the world for a little while in order to 'come home to ourselves'. In the busy work world, it can be extremely difficult to give priority to the attention that we need for ourselves.

> I enjoyed the meditation sessions we did in class and I would have loved to have kept up with it in some way, but it just didn't seem to happen for me. By the time I'm up in the morning, sorted the kids out, got ready for work, had a long day at work, then went to mother's to help my sister take care of her, well, meditation seemed the last thing on the list. I'm sure I'll get back to it someday, but right now I just have to get on with life as it is.

Stepping aside and having some time for ourselves, when there seem to be so many other pressures and priorities, can seem like an insurmountable obstacle. Of course, there could be some reasons why we continue with our packed lives: at one level it can be used as an excuse for not taking further action. Knowing inwardly that the spiritual path can be difficult, perhaps we may choose to stay with the status quo rather than engage in something that is full of uncertainty and possible difficulty. The following suggestions may be helpful:

- Join a group of other 'searchers' – perhaps a meditation group at a local college, a nearby church or other religious group with whom you feel comfortable (but keep in mind the cautions we discuss about gurus and groups in Chapter 5).
- Set up a group, perhaps at work or in your neighbourhood, of like-minded colleagues.
- Develop a plan of care for yourself that is realistic for you (see Chapter 3) and which does not cause you to give up because you have asked too much of yourself. For example, if an hour of exercise or meditation every morning and afternoon is not possible in your circumstances, then reduce the time and frequency to a pattern that suits you. It can only be disheartening if you set unrealistic goals, so find an approach that works for you, even a few minutes each day can be beneficial – perhaps five minutes at lunchtime being alone and quiet and/or a short walk each evening.
- Make that time for personal space that you always promised yourself. It is not necessary, as we will discuss in more detail in the Chapter 5, to

disappear into the hills of Tibet to a remote Làmasery to gain spiritual insight. Some people have the opportunity to do this, but for most of us it is not possible. Indeed, as we have suggested already, much of what we need for our spiritual work may be present in our lives already, without us being aware of it. A period of retreat, repeated at regular intervals, perhaps a week or a day or two every year, an occasional weekend, or whatever can be fitted realistically within your schedule will be helpful.

• Be easy on yourself. If your desire for more consistent inner work cannot be met at present, there is nothing wrong in putting it on the back burner for a little while until the time seems right for you.

We have a long history in the Trust of providing team away–days, planning weekends and so on for executive staff. Eventually, the message got through that those working at clinical level needed it too. We began to develop team-building and relaxation sessions for staff over 2 or 3 days. The evaluations have been highly positive, whether the days have been structured or not, or whether there has been a specific goal or piece of work to do or not, that time off-site, with colleagues, with a supportive facilitator, with someone to care for and feed them for a change, has enormously increased motivation and commitment at work. People have returned re-energised and far more positive in their work. There are signs that this has reduced sickness and absenteeism levels as well.

More enlightened employers are paying more attention to the needs of their staff in ways like this, as we suggested in Chapter 3. Where there is no provision at work, it may mean seeking out facilities and networking locally or nationally, locating like-minded groups of others. Carers at home may find that they can be helped by respite facilities provided by voluntary organisations or local hospitals and hospices. When the one we are caring for can be cared for by others for a little while, it gives us time to rest and renew our strength. It may be possible to take advantage of this time to find a place for quiet recuperation; even better if there are activities that can be done, e.g. learning meditation, praying with others, taking a sauna or having a massage, and we can subsequently integrate the effects of these activities into our daily lives.

More challenging is to stay with that stillness and sense of peace we can gain in retreat, be it for minutes, days or weeks, and hold it in our everyday lives. This is where developing a regular practice and routine will help. For some, it might be a daily session of exercise or meditation, for others, a regular visit to church or a weekly therapy group. In this way it may be possible to build the idea of sanctuary – sacred time and space for ourselves with or without specific spiritual work being done – into the normal pattern of life.

The weekend retreat was a brilliant event, and in the grounds of the farm we regularly used the 'sanctuary' for meditation and prayer. Some of the groupwork was held in there. It was a lovely room, set out with comfortable cushions and with a soft light. There were times set aside when it was for silent meditation only. I like the idea of being able to go to a certain place and be still and quiet at

> regular intervals. It was wonderful to have all that peace and relaxation, but the trouble is, after a few days back in the old routine, you seem to be back at square one. There needs to be some way of keeping it going beyond the retreat.

This idea of 'keeping it going' is an important one, and we will develop some further suggestions along these lines in the concluding chapter. If, as we have suggested, work and the strain of being with those needing care is a major cause of stress, then it would seem advantageous to set up a sanctuary in the workplace. This may be anything from a small corner at home or in the office as indicated above, to creating a special place for retreat, even if it is only for a few minutes. Those who have become well grounded in caring for themselves and have deepened, for example their meditation practice, may find that the need for time away from the caring context gets less and less. Learning to detach from the big drama so that it does not drain us, yet remaining actively involved in the world, is an ability reported by those who profoundly deepen their spiritual practice. And these are not supermen or women; they have just committed themselves to a certain path that enables them to work effectively in the pain and suffering of the world without it causing catastrophic stress or burnout for themselves.

One group of healthcare workers we have worked with has developed its own sanctuary in the hospital. Apart from a labyrinth and individual sacred spaces in offices and wards, a room was set aside as a staff sanctuary. Closed to the public, the room is softly decorated and furnished with chairs set in a circle, a candle and flowers in the centre. It is non-denominational, and no food, talking or smoking, are permitted there. There are guidance notes on how to use the room, which is kept open 24 hours a day, and staff can enter and be silent, pray or meditate there at any time. A few books of inspiring literature are available, and a training programme in meditation for hospital staff coincided with its creation. Telephone numbers of the hospital chaplain, independent counsellor and other helplines are on display to encourage those who need it to seek further help. Creating a sanctuary at home or in the workplace is possible. The most important place to create it, however, is within ourselves. Then the suffering in the world does not drag us down, for within ourselves we have found and can remain in that sacred space where we are always safe. A room or a retreat can be sanctuary, but the most important sanctuary we can learn of exists within.

COMPLEMENTARY THERAPIES

There is a growing advocacy for the integration of the complementary therapies into mainstream healthcare, and many people see them as part of holistic and spiritual care (Featherstone & Forsyth 1997, Foundation for Integrated Medicine 1997). Spiritual care is an integral part of holistic healthcare. Benson (1996) found that almost one-quarter of patients reported feeling 'more spiritual' after relaxation exercises and that they experienced fewer medical symptoms than those who reported no sense of spirituality.

A relaxation response is commonly reported with a great many complementary therapies. Furthermore, it seems that the patient is not the only one to gain, but the caregiver does too. Studies into almost all the therapies report beneficial effects for the caregiver as well as for the care receiver (Sayre-Adams & Wright 1995, Woodham & Peters 1998) The complementary therapies may be having a healing effect additional to that from the various substances and techniques used because of the fact that their methodology requires time to be taken and personal attention given, usually on a one-to-one basis.

Complementary therapies have become much more popular in recent years, some studies indicating that up to half the population in some European countries such as the UK now visit a complementary therapy practitioner each year (Woodham & Peters 1998). Until recently, much of orthodox medical practice has kept the complementary therapies at arm's length, arguing that their research base was inadequate. The volume of good-quality research available now, not least that covered by Woodham & Peters' survey, makes this argument less tenable. Woodham & Peters further comment that:

In holistic medicine, spiritual concerns rank with those of mind and body. We are creatures who puzzle over what life means, where we come from and where we are bound. To be anxious and bewildered at times is to be human. For many of us, the past has been painful, the present insecure and the future uncertain. In the struggle to make sense of life, certain activities create a supportive framework that connects us to our inner selves, to each other and to the world. These activities include art, literature, music, community, family, worship and play and they are especially important when illness presents us with the reality of vulnerability, limitations and dependency. Broadly speaking, this is the realm of spirituality.

As a TT [Therapeutic Touch] practitioner for several years, I have become very clear about one thing. I get as much out of it as my clients do. There is a connection between us when I am at work that transcends the treatment. We are both in a place that feels whole, relaxed, at one with each other. This is part of its mystery to me, and as I have become more expert in my practice, so too have I become more in awe of the healing process and of where it might come from. I am sure it is not me that is doing the healing. I am sure that it is not something passing though or around me. It is more an opening, to a knowledge and acceptance of something that is already there, and by working with people in the way that I do, I am convinced that it is the coming together and the being available for healing that allows the healing to happen. This has inspired me to deepen my own awareness and practice of my spirituality – through prayer, contemplation, going to church and meditation. It has also made me make sure that I put myself in a place of healing as well – I receive TT from a fellow practitioner, and make a point of having an aromatherapy massage on a regular basis.

It is not in the scope of this text to advocate or give details about any particular therapy for caregivers or care receivers. What we do suggest is that the therapies have a part to play as healing arts in helping us and those we care for along the spiritual journey, towards right relationship. The texts that we have mentioned provide excellent introductions to the many therapies, together with contact points, how to make choices and the up-to-date research base. We strongly recommend that any reader who has not already done so investigate one of the reputable therapies as an aid to personal and spiritual support, deepening one's understanding of the healing process. And, where appropriate, consider undertaking training in a particular therapy to integrate it into an existing caring role.

SHAMANISM

Imagination has always been an integral part of the healing process. Until the dawning of the scientific age, those who were able to help others with the powers of the imagination were given the highest place in the healing hierarchy (Achterberg 1985). Now with the increase in mind–body medicine and people's longing for things spiritual or transpersonal, naturalistic practices are returning, many of them being reintroduced by nurses and other healthcare professionals.

Imagery, or imagination, affects the body intimately on both mundane and profound levels. A lover's scent calls forth the biochemistry of emotion. A mental rehearsal of an interview evokes muscular change, blood pressure elevation, brainwave changes and sweat gland activity. A paralyzed patient makes a pilgrimage to Lourdes, a person with cancer journeys to Mexico for an unproven treatment, a witch doctor shakes the bones and utters a curse. Patients everywhere are administered placebos and relief from pain, nausea, anxiety or even a decrease of tumor cells occurs. As well as an attitude and perhaps a physical change, their biochemistry actually undergoes a transformation. (Dossey 1993)

Achterberg (1985) cites a story of the cardiologist, Bernard Lown, who told of a critically ill patient whose cardiac muscle was irreparably damaged, and for whom all therapeutic means had been exhausted. During his rounds, the doctor commented to his colleagues, and this was heard by the patient, that the patient's heart had a 'wholesome gallop'. To a cardiologist this means that the heart is about to fail. The patient recovered, however, and was discharged home. Later, at the outpatient clinic, the patient told Dr Lown that he knew what had made him better – the knowledge that he had a 'gallop'. This was interpreted by the patient as meaning that he must have a lot of 'kick' to his heart and therefore could not be dying. He knew instantly that he would recover! Achterberg notes that the words, conveying to the patient an image of a horse that still had 'kick' to it, were believed to have shifted the patient's perception from one of illness and negativity into one of health and positivity.

Exciting research has been pursued by Candace Pert (1997) on the mind–body connection. Whole new vistas of the nature of health and healing have opened up as a result. Chopra (1997) notes how our neuropeptides and their receptors are the 'actual biological underpinnings of our awareness, manifesting themselves as our emotions, beliefs, and expectations and profoundly influencing how we respond to and experience our world'. He believes that this research validates what 'shamans, rishis, and alternative practitioners have known and practiced for centuries ... the body is not a mindless machine – the body and mind are one'. This profound relationship between all the parts of our body, mind and soul seems to be accessible and can be nourished by such therapies as imagery, hypnosis, biofeedback and Therapeutic Touch (TT).

The work of the shaman, in a modern sense, is done in this 'imaginary' realm. A definition of a shaman is one who journeys into another reality (or dimension) at will, a state of consciousness conducive to special problem-solving abilities, in order to gain information to help or heal an individual or a community. 'The limitations of time and space are transcended ... Rocks and stones speak. Men turn into animals and animals into men. It is a world replete with archaic symbolism, in which the shaman journeys the breadth of the universe or around the moon on missions of utmost importance to his people' (Kraus, cited in Achterberg 1985).

Shamans are characterized as priests, physicians, magicians, sorcerers, exorcists, political leaders, and mountebanks by Mircea Eliade (1964), an author of classic anthropological and theological works who has reviewed the vast amount of literature on shamanism. The state of consciousness that a shaman enters by means of sound, movement or the taking of sacred substances is one of ecstasy or trance, which is a highly specific, special category of altered state, and we do not wish to imply that anyone can be a shaman or do shamanic acts (Sayre-Adams 1996). However, as the words and concepts are now being interpreted in popular culture, shamanism relates to the practice of any sort of non-medical, folk or mentalistic healing, or to any health system that does not incorporate western medicine.

A shaman may be a medicine man or a witch doctor, but very few medicine men or witch doctors are shamans, for the shaman's path is first and foremost a spiritual one. Shamans are technicians of the sacred and only rarely concern themselves with the physical. They believe that all illness comes from the patient's soul losing its power – a soul loss (Ingerman 1991) – and their way of healing involves reuniting the soul with the body, which then is empowered to heal itself.

Many healthcare professionals have found the concepts of shamanism or working in the realms of the imaginary to be an exciting, authentic and powerful way; a path that empowers them, helps them into right relationship with themselves and their inner work and allows them to participate more fully in life. As Achterberg (1985) observes, 'There is drama, here, as the elusive mysteries of the human mind begin to unfold – drama unparalleled on the battle field, or in space, or in politics, or in any other arena. The scientific paradigm shifts, the metaphors blend. It is a good time to be alive'.

SONG, MOVEMENT AND DANCE

> As waves upon my head the circling curl,
> So in the sacred dance weave and whirl.
> Dance then, O heart, a whirling circle be.
> Burn in this flame – is not the candle He?
>
> *Rumi (trans. Moyne & Barks 1994)*

Music has been a vital part of all societies and cultures, no matter how primitive or advanced they have been labelled. It is used in spiritual ceremonies and in celebrations. Armies march to battle with music, and mothers lull their infants to sleep with song. Music is played during rites of initiation, during funeral ceremonies, and on harvest and feast days. There is something about the power of music that cannot be expressed in verbal language. (Guzzetta, cited in Dossey et al 1988)

Scientists mapping the activity of the brain are beginning to unravel the reasons for the universal human response to rhythm and tone (Robertson 1996).

Closely allied to the complementary therapies and meditation are various movement techniques that are known to quiet the mind, aid concentration and focus on our inner selves, as well as helping to keep us physically fit. These include yoga, t'ai chi and chi qung. All of these approaches, while differing in technique, have a meditative and spiritual quality to them, a tendency to help us feel grounded, quiet the mind and come home to ourselves, aiding right relationship with our inner world through right relationship with our bodies. Many people report similar effects from everyday activities, usually classed as sports, such as swimming, climbing, hill walking and running.

Devotional singing and chanting have been used throughout human history as a means of promoting healing, elevating the spirits and to connect with each other and the divine. As suggested above, music and song can be used as part of a meditative process or to change the nature of the environment. A popular form of devotional singing, apart from those commonly used in religious services, with groups springing up all over the country, comes from Taizé. Turnbull (1997) writes that Taizé is the name of a religious order established in central France.

The brothers have created a body of music which can be sung in unison, in rounds, in harmonies. The songs are musically simple and consequently accessible to everyone. They are mostly written in Latin, being as it is a root language for many people who travel to Taizé. The songs are commonly written in minor keys, so they are more naturally inward and reflective in effect, rather than outgoing and exuberant, as is the case with traditional church hymns which are generally written in major keys. The sublime power of this shared devotional music is such that within about twenty minutes, a disparate group of women and men, essentially strangers to each other, become an intimate company of human beings, unified by the experience of connecting with the spiritual aspect of our human nature.

Of the 20 or so people in the chapel, I knew only one, and as this was my first experience of Taizé singing, I was doubtful that it was going to work. We were led gently into each song and a remarkable series of events occurred. First of all, people not used to singing with each other seemed to move very quickly into natural harmony. I was surprised to find that as we broke off into tenor and bass and other sections, we did not fall into chaos or go out of tune. A natural rhythm seemed to emerge, both to keep the songs going, and to all sing more quietly or loudly together. There was no conductor, no one to tell us when to harmonize or sing softly or loudly, and no one to tell us when to stop each song, yet when the moment came, we all just did, because it just felt right and everyone seemed to know it simultaneously. The chapel seemed to vibrate with a gentle energy of its own afterwards, and we all stood there for what seemed like an age in the silence, each one of us lost in our own reverie. I felt utterly calm, relaxed and at one with God and those people.

Bringing song into the caring relationship has many possibilities and there is an increasing interest in the use of sound for healing. Music produces alterations in the physiology of the body.

Soothing music can produce a hypometabolic response characteristic of relaxation in which autonomic, immune, endocrine, and neuropeptide systems are altered. Music is nonverbal in nature and appeals to the right hemisphere, whereas traditionally, healthcare professionals use of verbalization has its primary effect on the logical left brain. Music therefore provides a means of communication between the right and left brain: (Beebe 1979)

The same sort of effect can arise through dance, and dance movement therapy evolved in the USA in the 1940s as a method of expressing thoughts and feeling through movement. Sacred dance, sometimes known as 'circle dancing' is derived mainly from the folk traditions of Europe. Turnbull (1997) describes them as being:

... usually circular in form, fairly disciplined and repetitive. Their appeal is that in the process of dancing, inner qualities such as harmony or joy or reverence, which are implicit in the music and the form of the movements, become evident to the group. As with our singing, intellectual considerations fall away, and participants have an inward sense of well-being, as much as a sense of sharing in the ambient consciousness of the group.

The intention of dance such as this is not to create polished performances, but to meet in harmony and community, where the movements follow a rhythm that grows from the group, creating a sense of coordination and oneness.

'Song and dance' writes Turnbull, 'are instinctive, accessible, inexpensive, suitable for young and old, part of our wellness and wholeness'. Circle dancing (and perhaps its more popular and fashionable cousin, line dancing, which lacks the same communal circular oneness but is also reliant upon united movement in given rhythms) is slowly being restored to popularity. Its close cousin, folk dancing, has remained an important part of much of European indigenous culture – movement, harmony and rhythm serving to

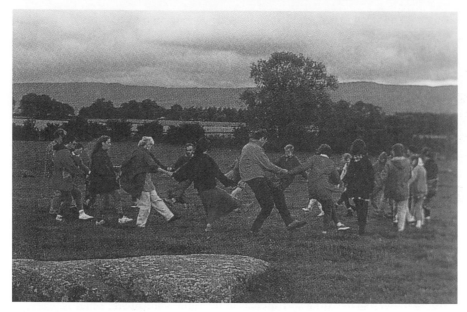

Figure 4.10 The power of the dance to bring people together. © Forder & Forder, reprinted with permission.

mark rites of passage and bind communities together. Sacred circle dance has increased enormously in popularity in recent years. Teachers and groups are present in many towns and cities, available both to the general public and to healthcare institutions. Organisations such as the Hart Centre offer teaching and guidance across the UK and abroad. Frances & Bryant-Jefferies (1998) believe that anyone can learn to dance (even those who are firm in their belief that they cannot) and write 'this is the power of the dance – to bring people together, to create harmony among a group of near strangers. Many aspects of modern life seem to separate us from each other, these dances encourage a renewed sense of community'. It seems that song and sacred dance are yet other gifts available to us both to reduce stress and as a path towards right relationship (Figure 4.10). Bernhard Wosien (cited in Frances & Bryant-Jefferies 1998), who has probably done more than any other individual to collate and reinvigorate sacred dance across Europe, believes this. Of sacred dances he writes 'One has to dance them to be totally present to discover their meaning and healing power. Only then does the religious origin reveal itself – the way to Oneness, from separation to community to vibrant togetherness'.

THE PATH OF SYMBOLISM AND MYTH: TAROT, I CHING, FAIRYTALES AND DREAMS

'One thing that comes out in myths is that at the bottom of the abyss comes the voice of salvation. The black moment is the moment when the real message of transformation is going to come. At the darkest moment comes the light' wrote the mythologist Joseph Campbell (1986). He believed that 'myths and symbols, by our recognition of what has meaning in them, show us our own states of unity, plurality and universality, and also function as agents of affirmation or negation and limitation dependent upon the meaning that we place upon them or the sense of recognition experienced at the moment in time.'

The abundant myths and symbols reflected in the Tarot 'represent the universal principles and processes that each human being, regardless of cultural imprinting or family conditioning, will experience at different times in his or her life and in different arenas of life' (Arrien 1987). Arrien notes how Carl Jung saw these principles and processes as the 'archetypes of the collective unconscious'. The Tarot, dreams, the I Ching, fairytales and storytelling can all help us tune into the collective unconscious.

'Creative ideas, in my opinion, show their value in that, like keys, they help to "unlock" hitherto unintelligible connections of facts and thus enable man to penetrate deeper into the mystery of life' (von Franz 1982). This quote of von Franz prompted Arrien to develop her work with the Tarot and to write:

… symbols may well be the creative ideas that function as a universal language in that area where an individual's internal and external worlds intersect and attempt to dialogue with one another. In any kind of inner work, whether it be in dreams, meditation, contemplation, guided imagery, or creative visualizations, symbols appear to us as signposts, or keys and they function as containers, revealers, or concealers of meaning to enable us to penetrate deeper into the mystery of life. (Arrien 1987)

Through Vaughan's (1979) influence, Arrien was inspired to look at the Tarot as a tool that could acknowledge and awaken an individual's intuitive processes. This then led Arrien to come to the conclusion that the Tarot is a 'symbolic map of consciousness and an ancient book of wisdom that reveals to us visually and symbolically the creative ideas and states of consciousness that appear in multiple existence in all cultures'. It is a 'visual map of consciousness and a symbolic system that offers insight into professional contribution, personal motives, and spiritual development of each individual'. Arrien has taken this ancient symbolic tool out of the realm of the fortune teller and placed it into the realm of personal development. The symbols on the Tarot speak to each person individually, according to the particular state of consciousness and understanding at that moment.

Although I had been interested in the Tarot for a long time, ever since I read a novel by Charles Williams where the Tarot had featured, the first time I encountered it was when a teacher introduced it to me. She made it very clear that the Tarot is best used as a meditative and developmental tool and used it this way with me. My 'life time' symbols turned out to be the Sun and the Wheel of Fortune. It so happened that in 'visions' experienced 5 years earlier both of these symbols had been experienced in a terrifying way. It was both extraordinary and ultimately reassuring as I came to know the friendly aspects of these cards and the ways one could work with the truths behind them. I was very attracted by the Thoth deck, which is visually beautiful in terms of colour and design. Having bought my own set, I bought Arrien's *Tarot Handbook: Practical Applications of Ancient Visual Symbols*, to go with it. Jung's ideas on synchronicity interested me, and the Tarot seemed to act in such a way as to synchronise the turn of the cards with the external events in my life. Up until now, accessing my interior world has never come easily to me, as I had always experienced it as dark and frightening. By using the Tarot, however, I have found an ideal tool to reflect back to me in an active, non-threatening way. Even the challenge cards are given a positive twist in Arrien's perceptive guide. I use the Tarot daily when possible, and over time some of the cards appear much more often than others. Using it daily like this one simply adopts a reflective and receptive attitude towards whatever emerges, having first thought about the day ahead, or the day that has just gone by. The imagery and symbolism are beginning to take hold of my imagination and I am beginning to recall the images spontaneously. The Tarot has given me a sense of security as I seek insight and meditational skills.

Using the Tarot as 'an outer mirror for internal and external processes aligns with the basic functions of mythology, or the essential services that mythology provides for human growth and development, and as a resource for self-revelation and self-reclamation processes' (Arrien 1987)

The I Ching or Book of Changes, one of the Five Classics of Confucianism, which provided a common source for both Confucianism and the Taoist philosophy, has exerted a living influence in China for 3000 years. Interest has been spreading in the west during the last few decades and it is increasingly being used in much the same way as the Tarot or dreams, in order to get in touch with the symbolism of the unconscious (Wilhelm 1950).

Pert (1997) suggests that 'dreams are just one more way God whispers in our ear, delivering messages to us via the psychosomatic network'. People have been dreaming and listening to dreams since the beginning of time; from Joseph's prophetic dreams in the Bible to the incubation of dreams widely used in the ancient temples of Greece. In the latter, priests and priestesses would help the dreamer to prepare for sleep by observing certain rituals which would encourage healing or problem solving in their dream temples. This is not so different from the modern version of taking our dreams to a Jungian therapist who uses them to help us heal and solve problems.

Some tribal people believe that the dream world is the real world and our reality is the dream (Bryant 1971). They see dreams as existing beyond time and space, in other dimensions. Jung's concept of the collective unconscious or Rogers' (1990) concept of pandimensionality would be the closest our own culture comes to an explanation of the timeless space of dreaming. Pert (1997), the brillant scientist, whose recent work has shown that it is our emotions that establish the crucial link between the body and mind, believes dreams to be 'direct messages from your bodymind, giving you valuable information about what's going on physiologically as well as emotionally,' and are a way of 'eavesdropping on the conversation that is going on between *psyche and soma* and of accessing levels of consciousness that are normally beyond awareness'.

Dreams are an easily accessible, gentle, personal thing to use as a path for inner knowledge of ourselves. Once we have made the committment to remembering our dreams, they will start to speak to us and will become clearer over time. Mallon (1987) suggests some ways in which we can begin to use our dreams for healing:

Keep a notebook or a tape recorder by your bed so that when you wake from a dream you are able to record it. Most of you will find writing more convenient and you should prepare for the dream by writing down the date before sleeping and then report the dream in as much detail as you can as soon as you wake. Don't worry about neatness, don't censor the material, and don't think you'll remember it later because it is such a brilliant dream – lots of dreams get lost that way! Get into the habit of keeping a dream diary and you'll find your rate of dreaming and recall will increase dramatically. Later, fill in any further details and see what you associate with the dream. Does it relate to anything happening in your waking life? How do you feel about it? Were you active or passive in the dream? Who were important figures? Who do the dream characters remind you of? Why should they appear now? What would you like to change? How does it fit in with other dreams, does it show development and progress? What is the message of the dream?

When you have been recording your dreams for some time you will find certain patterns occuring and will be able to build up your own unique dictionary of dream symbols. You will also learn which dreams warrant special attention, for instance warning dreams or diagnostic dreams. This will enable you to react appropriately to your own dream messages.

The most important parts of a dream are the feelings and emotions that accompany it, and it is essential to pay particular attention to these. As Mallon suggests, we too have found that usually with a little practice you can begin to understand your dreams and their content. Books on dreams and symbols should be used only as guides and not for seeking definitive interpretations. Dreams contain much archetypical material as myths and symbols, but the pattern of dreams and their interpretation must be uniquely our own. Likewise, it is necessary to be cautious when others suggest interpretations of our dreams, for no one can tell us what they mean to us – that must be for ourselves to decide. Self-interpretation is probably the most accurate; books and teachers can only suggest.

Marie-Louise von Franz (1982), a student of Carl Jung and a Jungian analyst, believes that 'fairy tales are the purest and simplest expression of collective unconscious psychic processes'. She goes on to say that they 'represent the archetypes in their simplest, barest and most concise form and it is this pure form of the archetypal images that afford us the best clues to the understanding of the processes going on in the collective psyche'. In myths or legends, or any other more elaborate mythological material, the 'basic patterns of the human psyche are overlaid with cultural material. According to Jung's concept, every archetype is in its essence an unknown psychic factor and has no possibility of translating its content into intellectual terms, whereas a fairytale's meaning is contained in the totality of its motifs connected by the thread of the story'.

I watched the documentary about Mother Theresa at work, and was so moved I had this tremendous urge to go out and join her. My family were panicked when I told them. At work, my colleagues thought I had finally gone crazy. I don't quite know why, but somehow what was going on out there seemed more important than what I was doing here. The suffering seemed greater. I felt I could do something. Something unique. I went through all kinds of plans in my imagination. Turning up in Calcutta to be welcomed with open arms, helping the dying like some sort of angel. After a little while, I woke up, as if I'd been in a dream. It felt just like that. One of my patients died while I was off duty, and the family came in to thank me. I thought 'Why? She was young, she had everything to live for, they should have been enraged with me at their loss'. But they just kept thanking me, saying how we didn't appreciate all that we had done, all the little kindnesses, the attention to their loved one in her last hours. It began to dawn on me after they had left, how little I valued what I already do. How what to me had become commonplace and ordinary was hugely important to those who receive it. I don't know why we don't always value what we are doing already. Maybe it's the 'grass is always greener' thing.

Valuing our own work of caring and recognising its sacred nature is perhaps the most important thing we can do towards restoring the sacred to caring. What we do is significant, it matters, and coming to accept that when we so often undervalue the contribution we make is part of the process of getting into right relationship. Our work provides us with the milieu for action in the world. Valuing it, being in right relationship with it, helps us toward right relationship with ourselves. The path of service, espoused throughout the ages as a holy path, is available to those of us who are carers right now should we choose it. Nurses, doctors, therapists – anyone in caring work is blessed, in that sense, by not having to go out and find work of compassionate service: they are in it already.

However, there is another perspective to this, from the point of view of the person receiving the care, as the following vignette illustrates:

I was a mess. Not only was I still in the midst of a four-year 'spiritual crisis' which had been fed by watching educational TV programmes about how old the earth was and how big the universe was, which made me aware of my own insignificance, but I had just had the laser surgery for my eyes that I had been dreaming of having for the past 20 years. Only it hadn't worked. I was one of the 10% who didn't get the anticipated benefits. I was blind some of the time and the other times my eyes were fluctuating so much that they were difficult to correct. This necessitated frequent contact with doctors. I'd had a long-standing dislike of doctors because, in spite of my extensive training to be a 'good patient', my previous contacts with doctors had left me feeling stupid and ugly – I felt they treated me with such disdain. Did I neglect to mention that I had been living and working in a casino in Las Vegas? Not exactly the ideal place for a person who was overly concerned with man's inhumanity to man, man's basic selfishness and of course, my inability to mobilize the energy to impact this, unlike all the other saints I had been reading or hearing about. On top of all this, I contracted pink eye. I went to three different doctors, only to get worse each day. After 10 days, eyes swollen shut and miserable, I called the emergency service (it was a

Saturday) of the doctor that had done my surgery. The doctor on call, a new one, called me back. I explained my symptoms and concerns and he wondered if I'd like to see him right away at his office. Being a good patient, I explained I just wanted reassurance that permanent damage was not being done to my eyes. He replied he was seeing another patient anyway and to come down. He changed the medicine I was putting in my eyes and told me to come back to see him the next day, and the next. I did. On Wednesday next, in the office, I had a profound, life-changing event. Waiting in the exam room, I was the last patient to be seen in what must have been an extremely busy day, as it was well past office hours. As I sat there, I heard this doctor with several other people and with each one there was such concern, interest and – dare I say it? – compassion in his manner with all of them. When he came to me, something – I can't say what – I can't put it in words – but something shifted and I felt I was in the presence of a great healer. And I felt healed. My sight hasn't returned but I'm no longer in despair. I now realise the impact one person can have. I cannot put into words the profound effect this had upon my psyche, my soul, my life.

THE PATH OF RELATIONSHIPS

Neal Walsch (1995) writes:

You have nothing to learn about relationships, you have only to demonstrate what you already know. There is a way to be happy in relationships and that is to use relationships for their intended purpose … relationships are constantly challenging; constantly calling you to create, express, and experience higher and higher aspects of yourself, grander and grander visions of yourself, ever more magnificent versions of yourself. Nowhere can you do this more immediately, impact fully and immaculately than in relationships. In fact, without relationships, you cannot do it at all.

Relationships provide us with the milieu to discover who we are by providing all the possible emotional experiences by which we can learn and expand our consciousness. Indeed, Newman (1986) has described health as 'expanding consciousness'. In relationships, we often see it as possible to find completeness with another. It might be more appropriate to see relationships as an opportunity for us to express our completeness.

If our work is part of our spiritual discipline, so are our relationships, the testbed for our spiritual awakening. What is the point of learning of love and compassion, of connectedness with the divine, if we cannot then ground that knowledge in our lives, our work and the people we relate to each day? Relationships provide us with the opportunity to 'walk our talk' – put into practice what we preach about spirituality. As we shall see in Chapter 5, the measure of a great spiritual teacher can be found not so much in the powerful words he speaks, but in how he treats his partner, family and friends.

James Jones (1996) remarks that this does not mean that all relationships must be in a state of constant connectedness and harmony:

Through the process of joining and separating again and again we learn to establish our identity in relation to others. The ebb and flow of closeness and distance maintains the dynamic balance between autonomy and connection. Times of separation undergird our individuality; times of connection keep us related to those around us.

In much of western culture, we are bombarded with signals which tell us that the only measure for a successful relationship is one of eternal bliss and happiness. If it is not working, then that gives us the reason to drop it and move on to the next one. 'One likes to believe that any trouble in a relationship is caused by outside circumstances, or the other partner. If only he or she would change, how perfect life would be!' note Pierrakos & Saly (1993). 'Yet in the landscape of our souls, the lower self and its effects also need to be discovered. Without facing what we least like about ourselves, we cannot understand why we do not have a well-working relationship, let alone make significant change.'

> My partner and I are so different. He thinks silently and logically for a long time, sorting out all the problems on the way until an idea becomes clear. Then he acts, quickly, decisively, lightening-like. I, on the other hand, have a glimmer and let each moment unfold, following what feels right, dreaming that glimmer into being, for days or even months before its form emerges. He likes order – a place for everything, everything in its place – I have to actually create chaos (if it isn't there already) out of which I can then be creative. We drive each other crazy. He tries to keep his impatience and anger under control and I try to keep my chaotic, watery self in check in order to be harmonious together. But then with his stress of 'walking on eggshells' in order to not upset me and my stress of being other than I am, one seemingly insignificant thing will cause one or the other of us to blow a fuse and we're off! But beneath it all – around and inside – is our deep spiritual connection, our love for one another and our deep knowingness and thanksgiving that God has given us each other in order to awaken. We'll sit and meditate for a while, alone or with each other, and that 'stuff' just melts away and we're back into right relationship. We are each other's spiritual practice.

Relationship is a high wire act. To the left is the irretrievable past – your personal history, your previous relationships, your triumphs and your grief, the momentum which mechanically seeks to repeat itself, your helplessness. To the right is the uncontrollable future – your expectations and fears, a thousand desires yet unfulfilled, fading dreams, your hopelessness … the tightrope is this present moment, this very instant in which we attempt to maintain some balance … when the balance is perfect, grace and disgrace dissolve equally into unconditional love. (Levine & Levine 1995)

Falling into unconditional love is falling into right relationship with another. Such unconditional love is a sacred act, for, believe Levine & Levine, it is not just embracing the beloved other person, it is embracing the Beloved, the divine, the sacred love.

It is interesting to consider also that our relationships are not just with people. If one facet of being in right relationship is the 'I-Thou' view (see Chapter 3), then this includes our relationship with all aspects of the world, including the plant and animal world. For many people, pets and other animals form their most significant, perhaps only, relationships. Indeed, pet therapy has emerged as a complementary therapy (Woodham & Peters 1998); from dogs and cats to dolphins and whales, animals have been involved in developing therapeutic relationships, especially with those who have a learning disability or communication difficulty. The comfort and pleasure we derive from keeping a pet, the responsibility of seeing to its welfare, these and other factors, as in all our relationships, are also teachers of right relationship.

Relationships, like all the other paths suggested in this chapter, have to be worked at. This does not necessarily mean that people in a relationship must remain forever together; the working at it may mean coming to the realisation that it is time to end the relationship as it is, if not end it all together. What this does mean is that we can see our work and relationships as grist for the mill. All the material we need to work on for our spiritual unfolding is right at our fingertips. Our marriages, partnerships, families, social contacts and our work are our spiritual discipline. Anyone who is in relationship and/or caring work, whether they acknowledge their spirituality or not, whether they have a practice such as meditation or movement or not, is accessing spiritual work. For such people to say 'I have no spiritual discipline' is therefore a contradiction in terms: if we are caring and in relationship, we have as much material for spiritual work available to us as any saint in a monastery or mystic in a retreat.

Thus far we have suggested a few gateways we can enter which lead to different paths for walking the inner journey. They are all paths of the heart, but to follow them safely we need guides: teachers, trusted colleagues and friends, inspiring literature, group and community opportunities, good therapists, counsellors and healers. They are all around us; there is no need to undertake the journey alone. When we are unsure of our guides, we can make a few tests to validate their authenticity, and we give some pointers to this in Chapter 5.

As to the paths themselves, only a few of the many hundreds of which we have explored here, it may be that they are relatively unimportant: the actual methods used may be secondary to the consciousness, the will, that we bring to them. They may work largely because we choose and make a commitment to them. We may often ask, where do I find my path, my teacher, be it a person or thing? Our teachers, whatever form they take – an event, a therapist, a relationship – tend to turn up when we are ready. Often, as we have suggested, they are right next to us, waiting to be discovered.

We have repeatedly used the metaphor of the pathway in this chapter, and the idea of a path suggests a journey, a movement forward from place to place in the physical world. Great literature on the spiritual journey from across the world has used a similar mechanism to describe our spiritual awakening. Very few of the paths we have suggested here actually require us to move from where we are. Our grist for the mill, our pilgrimage, does not require a retreat for 40 days and 40 nights into the desert or a long journey from continent to continent. Our pilgrimage is an internal one, a journey of adventure into the unknown to seek what we already really know in our hearts.

Most of us find it difficult to give up the ties and responsibilities of this reality. Our suggestion is that there is no need. The path for each of us is in the here and now. All we have to do is wake up to the possibilities, to open the doors before us, and walk through on a journey of discovery. The paths may be legion, but the destination is always the same, and it is Home.

REFERENCES

Achterberg J 1985 Imagery in healing; shamanism and modern medicine. Shambhala, Boston
Aldridge D 1996 Music therapy research and practice in medicine. JKP, London
Anderson R F 1992 How to draw or lay out a replica of the Chartres Cathedral Labyrinth. Unpublished information sheet, Sebastapol, California
Anderson S 1997 The Virago book of spirituality. Virago, London
Arrien A 1987 The Tarot handbook: practical applications of ancient visual symbols. Arcus, Sonoma
Artress L 1995 Walking a sacred path – rediscovering the labyrinth as a sacred tool. Riverhead, New York
Bachmann M O 1995 Influences on sick building syndrome symptoms in three buildings. Social Science and Medicine 40(2): 245–251
Beebe R 1979 Synesthesia with music. Dromenon 2 (Winter) 7. In: Guzetta C 1988 Music therapy: hearing the melody of the soul. In: Dossey B, Keegan L, Guzzetta C, Kolkmeir L 1988 Holistic nursing – a handbook for practice. Aspen, Gaithersburg
Benson H 1996 Timeless healing. Simon & Schuster, London
Biley F 1996 Hospitals: healing environments. Complementary Therapies in Nursing and Midwifery 2: 110–115
Brueton D 1997 Rehallowing our Sacred Land. Kindred Spirit 39 (Summer): 25–27
Bryant D 1971 The kin of Ata are waiting for you. Random House, New York
Caddy E 1971 And God spoke to me. Findhorn Press, Findhorn
Caddy E 1986 Opening doors within. Findhorn Press, Findhorn
Campbell J 1986 Inner reaches of outer space: metaphor as myth and as religion. St James Press, Toronto
Chetan A, Brueton D 1994 The sacred yew. Arkana, Harmondsworth
Chopra D 1997 Foreword. In: Pert C. Molecules of emotion. Scribner, New York
Dix A 1996 Is God good value? Health Service Journal 11th July: 24–26
Dossey L 1993 Healing words. HarperCollins, San Francisco
Dossey L 1996 Prayer is good medicine. HarperCollins, San Francisco
Dossey B, Keegan L, Guzzetta C, Kolkmeier L 1988 Holistic nursing – a handbook for practice. Aspen, Gaithersburg
Eliade M 1964 Shamanism: archaic techniques of ecstasy. Princeton University Press, New Jersey
Easwaran E (trans) 1988 The Upanishads. Arkana, London
Eliot T S 1943 Four Quartets. Harcourt Brace, Orlando
Featherstone C, Forsyth L 1997 Medical marriage. Findhorn Press, Findhorn
Forder E, Forder J 1995 The light within. Usha Publications, Cumbria
Foundation for Integrated Medicine 1997 Integrated healthcare. FIM, London
Frances L, Bryant-Jefferies R 1998 The sevenfold circle – self awareness in dance. Findhorn Press, Findhorn

Freshwater D 1997 Geopathic stress. Complementary Therapies in Nursing and Midwifery 3: 160–162

Harvey A 1994 The way of passion: a celebration of Rumi. Souvenir, London

Ingerman S 1991 Soul retrieval – mending the fragmented self. Harper, San Francisco

Johns C, Freshwater D 1998 Reflective practice. Blackwell, Oxford

Jones J 1996 In the middle of this road we call our life. HarperCollins, London

Kamalashila 1988 Sitting. Windhorse, Birmingham

Kitson A 1988 On the concept of nursing care. In: Fairbairn G, Fairbairn S (eds) Ethical issues in caring. Aldershot, Avebury

Ladouceur P (ed) 1996 Sacred words. Findhorn Press, Findhorn

Lawlor R 1995 Sacred geometry. Thames & Hudson, London

LeShan L 1974 How to meditate. Thorsons, London

LeShan L 1995 Mobilizing the life force, treating the individual. Conversation with Larry LeShan by Bonnie Horrigan. Alternative Therapies in Health Care Medicine 1995 1(1): 62–69

Levine S, Levine O 1995 Embracing the beloved. Doubleday, New York

Longaker C 1998 Facing death and finding hope. Arrow, London

Lonegrin S 1991 Labyrinths: ancient myths and modern uses. Gothic Image, Glastonbury

MacInnes E 1996 Light sitting in light. HarperCollins, London

Mallon B 1987 Women dreaming. Fontana Collins, London

Mann A T 1993 Sacred architecture. Element, Shaftesbury

Maxwell M, Tschudin V 1990 Seeing the invisible. Arkana, Harmondsworth

McCullogh L 1997 Where wonders settle. Common Boundary (Nov/Dec) 38–41

McLuhan T C 1996 Cathedrals of the spirit. Thorsons, London

Moyne J, Banks C 1994 Say I am you – a book on Rumi. Maypop, Athens

Murray E 1997 Cultivating sacred space. Pomegranate, Maldon

Newman M 1986 Health as expanding consciousness. Mosby, St Louis

Nightingale F 1859 Notes on nursing – what it is and is not. 1980 edn. Churchill Livingstone, Edinburgh

Ornish D 1998 Love and survival: the scientific basis for the healing power of intimacy. HarperCollins, New York

Osho 1995 What is meditation? Element, Rockport

Pakenham T 1996 Meetings with remarkable trees. Orion, London

Palmer M, Palmer N 1997 Sacred Britain. Piatkus, London

Pennick N 1996 Celtic sacred landscapes. Thames & Hudson, London

Pert C 1997 Molecules of emotion. Scribner, New York

Pierrakos E, Saly J 1993 Creating Union – the pathwork of relationship. Pathwork Press, Madison

Ram Dass, Bush M 1992 Compassion in Action. Bell Tower, New York

Robertson 1996 Music of the spheres. Independent on Sunday, 5 May

Rogers M 1990 Nursing; science of unitary, irreducible, human beings. In: Barrett E (ed) Visions of Rogers' science-based nursing. National League for Nursing, New York

Rossbach S 1992 Feng shui. Rider, London

St Teresa of Avila 1995 The interior castle. Fount, London

Sayre-Adams J 1996 Ancient shamanism and modern nursing. European Nurse 1(3): 187–193

Sayre-Adams J, and Wright S G 1995 The theory and practice of therapeutic touch. Churchill Livingstone, Edinburgh

Schroeder-Sheker T 1994 Music for the dying: a personal account of the new field of music thanatology. Journal of Holistic Nursing 12(1): 56–64

Soine L 1995 Sick building syndrome and gender bias; imperiling women's health. Social Work in Health Care 20(3): 51–65

Storr A 1996 Feet of clay. HarperCollins, London

Stoter D 1995 Spiritual aspects of health care. Mosby, London

Streep P 1997 Altars made easy. HarperCollins, London

Thurnell-Read J 1995 Geopathic stress. Element, Dorset

Turnbull I 1997 Conference report of Taizé singing and sacred dance. Sacred Space Foundation, Penrith

Vaughan F 1979 Awakening intuition. Anchor Press/Doubleday, New York

Vaughan F 1995 Shadows of the sacred. Theosophical Publishers, Wheaton

von Franz M L 1982 Interpretation of fairytales. Spring Publications, Dallas

von Pohl G F 1993 Earth currents: causative factors of cancer and other diseases. Frech-Verlag, Stuttgart

Walsch N M 1995 Conversations with God – an uncommon dialogue. Hodder & Stoughton, London

Wilhelm H 1950 Trans. Baynes C F The I Ching or Book of Changes. Bollingen Foundation, New York

Woodham A, Peters D 1998 Encyclopaedia of complementary medicine. Dorling Kindersley, London

Wright S G 1998 The reflective journey begins a spiritual journey. In: Johns C, Freshwater D 1998 Reflective Practice. Blackwell, Oxford

The shadows of the sacred

Know thyself.

Inscribed over the entrance to the oracle at Delphi

HIDING FROM THE DARK

In our search for the sacred, there is a common tendency to want blissful experiences, full of light and love, and to turn away from the mundane, the nasty or what we judge as darkness or evil. This applies to what we see as the darkness in ourselves as well as in the rest of the world. It is relatively easy to look at the wider world with all its shadows and pain; much more difficult to turn the roving eye inward and see what dark shadows may lurk within ourselves. However, if we are to enter into right relationship with others and the wider world, we must also embark upon that voyage of self-discovery to enter right relationship with ourselves which includes both the light and the shadow. Sometimes, what the ancients called 'the dark night of the soul' may be a spiritual emergency that precipitates a deeper spiritual search. Many, if not all, of the paths we discussed in Chapter 4, can potentially lead us into a recognition of our own darkness. We may be inclined to prefer the sweeter experiences, but when we see the darkness, it is important to remember that it, too, has teachings for us. When the shadow is embraced and integrated, we become whole, healed and, paradoxically, more energy, not less, is available to us.

Throughout the ages, in many spiritual teachings, from the Upanishads to the Bible, from the Sufi and Christian mystics of the middle ages to modern-day Buddhist teachers such as Thich Nhat Hanh, the same message is conveyed: that light and dark exist in all things, both are part of the One/the Creator/God, and that the union of the two forces through acceptance and compassion is a universal goal. In becoming individuated, that same goal for each human being presents itself – to work with not only the light and love in ourselves, but also our shadow side. Thich Nhat Hanh (1993) writes:

> I am the mayfly metamorphosing on the surface of the river.
> I am also the bird, which when spring comes, arrives in time to eat the mayfly.
> I am a frog swimming happily in the clear water of a pond.
> I am also the grass snake who, approaching in silence, feeds itself on the frog.
> I am the child in Uganda, all skin and bones, my legs as thin as bamboo sticks.

I am also the merchant of arms, selling deadly weapons to Uganda.
I am the twelve year old girl refugee on a small boat, who throws
herself into the ocean after being raped by a sea pirate.
I am also the pirate, my heart not yet capable of seeing and loving…
…my joy is like spring, so warm it makes flowers bloom in my hands.
My pain is like a river of tears, so full it fills up all the four oceans.

As joy and light are a part of life, so are darkness and suffering. The struggle with the darker part of ourselves is well illustrated in countless mystical texts and other writings about the inner journey. It forms part of the typical hero's journey in popular culture both ancient and modern, from Peresphone's journey into the underworld of Greek mythology to Luke Skywalker's struggle with himself in the Star Wars series. Such archetypes inform us of the nature of the endless human endeavour to balance the light and dark in each of us. This is beautifully illustrated not just in the stories of adult experience, but by the daily trials of children as they come to terms with right and wrong, desires, guilt, ingratitude, lust, envy, anger and so on. All the everyday tussles with the seven deadly sins and more, begin in our earliest awakenings in childhood. For example, in *Children's Letters to God* (Hample & Marshall 1992) we find children writing of their inner turmoil such as:

Dear God,
If we come back as something
please don't let me be
Jennifer Horton
because I hate
her.
Denise

or

Dear God,
Thank you for
the baby brother
but what I prayed
for was a puppy.
Joyce

or

Dear God,
That fairy you sent left 5 cents
for my tooth and a quarter for my brother's. So
you still owe me 20 cents
Peter

Dear God,
If you give me a genie lamp like Alladin I will give you anything you
want
except my money
or my chess set.
Raphael

At an early age, children exhibit a capacity to perceive the choices between
'good' and 'bad' that face them. Adults are often surprised and touched by
the compassion of children (often dismissed by the worldly wise as unrealistic
or naive) and their ability to see the world and its wrongs, and possible
solutions, in uncluttered and obvious ways.

At a recent conference, one of the speakers had been unable to attend
because of a serious illness. The evening before the conference began, a short
meditation took place to envision healing and wellbeing for the ill person.
Matthew Jack, attending the conference with his parents, was only two, and
he gazed bemused at the silent crowd enveloped in candlelight. In trying to
explain what was happening, he was told that 'we are all being quiet in
order to send good wishes to Larry to make him better'. Clearly struggling
with this strange idea, Matthew Jack decided that the adults were obviously
missing the point. The silence was broken as the voice of a child called out
'… woo, woo, woo, woo, woo, woo …' The sound of an ambulance being sent
to help the sick clearly made more sense to him as an example of good
intentions!

Ram Dass in his many teachings often tells the tale of his reflections and
meditations upon the many different, including the darker, parts of himself.
As he observed each of them as separate entities standing before him – the
parts of him that were the friend, the professor, the son; the parts that showed
lust, anger, despair, possessiveness and so on – he suddenly became aware
that, if they were all out there looking at him, then 'who's minding the store?'
In other words, these elements of ourselves, our ego, our personality, are not
us. Something else, deeper and more mysteriously aware, is both involved
with and stands apart from who we think we are.

As we come to witness all those parts of us that we have created and that
have been created for us down the years, we can begin to enter a new
relationship with the world. When we realise that we are not who we thought
we were, we can come to understand the real 'I' that exists beneath all those
constructs and ties to the personality. When we can relate to the real 'I' then
the power of who we thought we were is diminished. We emerge chicken-
like from an eggshell into a new perspective of who we really are. All the
darker parts of the self are but grist for the mill, teachers, things to work with
as we follow the road that leads to deeper understanding of the self. However,
so often we seek to bury our nastier side, attempting to hide it in the belief
that if ignored it will go away, or at least lose its influence over us. The

opposite seems to be the case. To do spiritual work, to discover the sacred within ourselves, we cannot bypass the emotional work. All the great spiritual teachers down through the ages sought not to bury their darker sides, but to work with them, suffer with them and bring them into the light.

However, for most participants in the search, the darkness in ourselves has become something to avoid. We have attended so many gatherings, meetings and 'New Age' events where everyone appears happy and shiny and smiley. However, the darkness could be sensed underneath. The light is but a front, placed like a mask over the face. David Steindl-Rast (1991) writes of the New Age searchers for whom 'The shadow has been conspicuous by its absence. Seekers often are led to believe that with the right teacher or the right practice, they can transcend to higher levels of awareness without dealing with the more petty vices or ugly emotional attachments'. He cites Colorado journalist Marc Barash (1993) who says 'Spirituality, as repackaged for the new age, is a confection of love and light, purified of pilgrimage and penance, of defeat and descent, of harrowing and humility'.

This does not mean that we have to deliberately plunge ourselves into a pit of danger and despair if we are to pursue our understanding of our spirituality. Nevertheless, the path should be approached with care and caution. *The Cloud of Unknowing* (Wolters 1978), believed to be a late 17th-century text on the spiritual journey by an unknown author, reminds us that we should 'be careful in this matter, and do not overstrain yourself emotionally or beyond your strength. Work with eager enjoyment rather than with brute force. The more eager your work, the more humble and spiritual it becomes'. Jesus, in the Gospel of St Thomas (Robinson 1988) urged 'Let him who seeks continue seeking until he finds. When he finds, he will become troubled. When he becomes troubled, he will be astonished, and he will rule over all'.

Making the 'trouble' a source of learning seems to be the object lesson in confronting the shadow in ourselves. Thus we become alchemists of the soul, transforming lead into gold. In the shadow there is hope.

ALCHEMY

The ancient art of alchemy (from the arabic *al kimiya* – the art of changing one substance into another) is often reduced to a view of strange men in even stranger clothes, dabbling in magic in an effort to turn lead into gold in pursuit of great riches. We need to look at the story as allegorical, of finding ways to turn the leaden parts of ourselves into the golden possibilities of illumination and awareness. The theme of alchemy is echoed in the Arthurian legends of the pursuit of the holy grail. Working with all the darkness of the world, the knights of the round table sought the chalice believed to have been used by the Christ himself. Again we can see allegory at work here, replicated in myths and stories around the world throughout the ages – the heroic journey into darkness to discover a great treasure. Perhaps the reward should be seen metaphorically, not so much as earthly riches or power but as self-discovery and enlightenment.

In his modern fable, *The Alchemist*, Paolo Coelho's (1993) heroic boy hears the whispering of his heart, which says: 'Be aware of that place where you are brought to tears. That's where I am, and that's where your treasure is'. The boy undertakes a courageous journey to discover his treasure, realising in the end that it was not gold or jewels, but himself. The alchemy of the spiritual quest concerns the search for the hidden treasure of ourselves, turning darkness into light. To do this, we need the courage to undertake our own hero or heroine's journey, seeking and becoming aware of the dark, transmuting it into light. Thus we find our treasure, our holy grail. Personal alchemy is turning the leaden parts of ourselves into gold. Such a transformation is integral to our own health, our own right relationship with ourselves and perhaps our God.

Such an alchemical process affects not just ourselves, but everything around us. As we shift our view of the world and our place in it, there is a knock-on effect in our work, our relationships, our interests and everything in our daily lives. As we turn more into light, others around us cannot avoid being affected by it. Coelho also writes that 'When we strive to become better than we are, everything around us becomes better too'. Andrew Harvey (1991) documenting his own spiritual awakening and especially his challenging contact with Mother Meera, adds 'No awakening can be personal or selfish. Every awakening spreads its power and light throughout the world'. Watson's (1980) report on the 'hundredth monkey' study is interesting. In this study, skills learned by a group of monkeys being studied by anthropologists were picked up by other groups without any physical or social contact between them. It seems that the other groups of monkeys somehow obtained the information from the first group once a critical mass of monkeys with the knowledge had been reached in the first group. Similar experiments have been conducted with other animals and it seems that by some process we do not yet fully understand when enough individuals shift their way of being in the world in some way, the rest follows automatically. The implications of this concept in regard to a mass of people awakening spiritually are enormous.

Thus the notion of our own work, healing and coming home to ourselves, of transforming darkness into light, has an impact upon others. In *The Garden of the Prophet*, Kahlil Gibran (1933) says: 'So shall the snow of your heart melt when the spring is come, and thus shall your secret run in streams to seek the river of life in the valley. And the river shall enfold your secret and carry it to the great sea …' In the spring, which comes shedding new light on our cold dark places, we melt to join the sum total of the conscious river of humanity. Our change makes a change in the whole.

THE DARK NIGHT OF THE SOUL

As we have suggested already, many of us involved in healthcare are ourselves struggling with the difficulties of relationships and the vagaries of our own personalities. It is acknowledged that we need to address the support of carers in terms of decent facilities, adequate help, knowledge, skills or rewards to continue caring. However, to become whole, there is also work that we have to do on ourselves, and this includes exploring our shadow side and dealing with our suppressed pain.

Throughout the ages, the mystical approach has documented the struggle that ensues in following the inner journey. The Christian mystical texts illustrate this well, from the writings of Hildegard of Bingen (Flanagan 1989) to St John of the Cross (1973), from the *The Cloud of Unknowing* (Wolters 1978) to *The Interior Castle* of St Teresa of Avila (1995). We find similar reports in the writings of the mystical sect of Islam, Sufism, such as Farud ud-din Attar's *The Conference of the Birds* (1984), in the Jewish Cabbalistic movement and in the Buddhist writings and so on. All such voyagers report on the extremes of pain and suffering that they experience as they go deep into themselves to discover the sacred.

For any seeker, whether connected to a religion or not, the inner journey has trials in store. An individual may not appear to have the hallmarks of a great mystic (Underhill 1911), but there is no doubt, as many sources report, that the journey is equally difficult and painful for all who undertake it. The methods or disciplines we choose to help us make this journey are many and varied, as we suggested in Chapter 4. All, however, are not pursued without some danger, as we shall see. This spiritual path, means that the participant takes personal risks, but as James Jones (1996) points out: 'Dangerous? Yes, but equally dangerous is a life without ecstasy, without the numinous, without depth, breadth, passion, meaning or purpose. Spirituality is process before content. Not memorising rules, facts or concepts, but freeing the mind and the heart to explore new worlds of insight'.

So, fear of the shadow side of ourselves, and of exploring it, will keep us from entering into right relationship (Figure 5.1). Yet it is contended throughout this text that being in right relationship in other areas of our lives is underpinned by right relationship with the self. Fear, however it manifests itself – as arrogance, braggadocio, bluster, avoidance or retreat – keeps us from deepening our understanding of ourselves. The poet and mystic, Rumi (1994) writes that though there are walls within and between us, there is hope, for there is always a 'window that opens'. That window may present itself in many forms – a sudden flash of insight, a personal trauma that shakes our view of the world, meeting a special teacher – whatever the cause, windows of opportunity regularly present themselves in our lives. Only our fear and ignorance keep us from recognising them.

Our egos, shored up by the endless wounds we have received in life, can make it difficult for us to risk the view through the window but look we must.

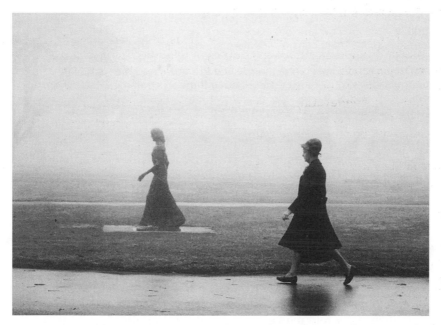

Figure 5.1 Exploring the shadow side of ourselves is part of right relationship. © Laurence Winram, reprinted with permission.

The path of life has left none of us unscathed or unwounded, and this applies no less to those involved in caring for others. As we suggested in Chapter 1, very large numbers of professional and informal carers are themselves 'co-dependent' or bringing their own difficulties into the caring relationship, however unconsciously. Healing the wounded healer is part of the work of those who seek to care for and heal others. As we move towards wholeness, we create the potential for those we care for to do likewise. In the New Testament, we are reminded of the charge which Jesus knew would be hurled at him because he sought to help others. Jesus expected his opponents, seeing him as a blaspheming madman, to tell him 'physician, heal thyself' before attempting to cleanse others. None of us is unwounded, yet our wounds can also be great teachers.

I got to the age of 40 and everything seemed to be falling apart, and all the stuff that wasn't – my job, my property, my opportunities – didn't seem to mean anything any more. The work I did in therapy, my taking up meditation, my spiritual search – often both painful and blissful – led me to look back on my life in different ways. I let go of the anger I had for my parents, about the lack of love and protection, about the betrayals and petty ignorances in my upbringing, about the violence and the abuse. Now I look back upon them, dare I say it, with gratitude. That is not to minimise their significance, or to make excuses for wrong behaviour. Rather, all those acts seem now to be so terribly well fitted in making up the jigsaw puzzle of who I am. They are part of the complete picture that is me. I do not regret them, not even the most horrific events, not now. I stand where I am now and look back upon them, they made me the richer, the more aware, the more compassionate man that I am. They helped me to get to this point of my life, and gave me the energy and insight to do the work that had to be done. No, I do not regret them. They are now just there, part of the wondrous interplay of forces that helped to forge this person: without them I would not have had the experiences I have had; without them I would not be who and where I am now, and I am content to be who and where I am now.

Turning darkness into light is demanding work. As Benjamin Franklin once said, there are three things that are extremely hard: 'Steel, a diamond and to know oneself'. However, much may depend on the way in which we look at it: a shift of perception may help us to see that a problem is not so great as we thought. There is an old story of a seeker, an inveterate smoker, who asks his Buddhist master 'Is it OK to smoke while I meditate?' 'Of course you must not!' replies the master, 'Nothing must distract you from your meditation practice in any way'. Somewhat cowed, he goes away and the next morning, while practising his walking meditation in the garden he sees a fellow novice smoking. 'Hey!' he calls out, 'The master told me quite clearly yesterday that we must not smoke while meditating'. 'That's strange', replied his fellow seeker. 'the master told me yesterday that it was quite all right to meditate while I smoke'.

Gandhi knew this struggle well when he said 'The only devils in the world are those running around in our own hearts. That is where the battle should be fought'.

A battle it may be, but it is not a war fought with weapons of destruction. We do not defeat darkness by using its own weapons against it. The more we fight, seek to repress or to destroy our pain, the stronger it grows. The weapons, if weapons they be, are not those that the darkness itself would use, but those of loving acceptance and understanding. In learning to love and accept all those parts of ourselves, all those experiences that we have hitherto seen as hateful or the memories of which we have sought to avoid, that is when they lose their power over us. Through loving acceptance, the power of darkness is turned to the power of light. The poet Wendell Berry (Zwieg & Abrams 1991) writes:

> To go in the dark with a light is to
> know the light.
> To know the dark, go dark.
> Go without sight, and find the dark, too,
> blooms and sings.
> and is travelled by dark feet and dark wings.

I was in a dark place, whether dream or nightmare or meditation, I don't know which. In this place I met a dark power who challenged me. I fought, oh how I fought. I hurled myself against it. Thrashed at it with a sword of gleaming light. I saw it fall, I retreated, only to see it grow again, each time stronger than before. I saw myself in heroic light, fighting the forces of evil to save the world; each time I crushed it or broke it, it would reassemble, more terrifying than before. At the last, I fell in exhaustion, dark hands clawing at me and folding me ever more tightly in their grip … I fell, surrendered, let go, prayed for help to all those who had helped me, Ram Dass, Mother Meera, Jesus, God … and in surrender came the light and I was back. That vision, image, whatever it was, lasted all night, and it was filled with fear. But I learned from it, I learned about myself, where my own darkness and weaknesses lay. I learned how the darkness itself works. In responding to me it revealed itself to me, as I too revealed something of me to myself. In knowing, the power of the darkness is lessened.

Carl Jung (1959) wrote of the 'collective unconscious', bringing it into common parlance. If we accept this concept, then there are implications beyond ourselves if we turn darkness to light. We may affect the sum total of darkness at work in the world. Some believe that there is an independent source of evil, a greater darkness that has a will of its own. James Hillman (1996) notes that: 'Behind the repressed darkness and the personal shadow – that which has been and is rotting and that which is not yet and is germinating – is the archetypal darkness, the principle of not-being, which has been named and described as the Devil, as Evil, as Original sin, as death, as Nothingness.' Whatever the answer to this question, over which scholars and mystics have pondered for centuries, it seems that what we can know is our own personal shadow. That part of the whole is given to each of us to work with. Rumi (1994) again reminds us that 'if thou hast not seen the devil, look at thine own self!' The notion of each of us contributing to the diminution of the darkness by working on ourselves is repeated by Robert Bly (1991) who says:

So the person who has eaten his shadow spreads calmness and shows more grief than anger. If the ancients were right that the darkness contains intelligence and nourishment and even information, then the person who has eaten some of his or her shadow is more energetic as well as more intelligent.

Ken Wilber (1991) reminds us that:

In this war between opposites, there is only one battleground – the human heart. And somehow, in a compassionate embrace of the dark side of reality, we become bearers of the light. We open to the other – the strange, the weak, the sinful, the despised – and simply through including it, we transmute it. In so doing, we move ourselves toward wholeness.

Thus from many viewpoints we can arrive at the same conclusion. Exploring our shadow side is an essential precursor to right relationship. It is not a task to be undertaken lightly, but the potential rewards of the work are immense. Furthermore, the status quo is not an option. Sooner or later in this life, if not, perhaps, in the next, we must come face to face with our own shadows. Jesus, in the Gospel of St Thomas (Robinson 1988), said 'If you bring forth what is within you, what you bring forth will save you. If you do not bring forth what is within you, what you do not bring forth will destroy you'.

To complicate matters, there are many blind alleys along the way. We need to be alert to them as summarised in the following seven sections.

1. SPIRITUAL MATERIALISM

Becoming attached to our spiritual progress may itself become a stumbling block, as can attachment to many of the tools we use on our journey or in our work. Such materialism ranges from a feeling that we cannot meditate, for example, unless certain precise conditions are met, to a deep attachment to wanting to become enlightened. Thus, the very desire for something such as enlightenment or deeper awareness can itself prevent these things coming about. For example, being enlightened includes giving up wants and desires, thus wanting and desiring enlightenment itself blocks us reaching that state. Mystics and spiritual teachers throughout the ages have warned their pupils of this trap. Furthermore, we can very easily become stuck in one particular element of our journey, or the desire for new experiences, or the wish to be more 'spiritually advanced' than others. The Buddhist saying, 'If you meet Buddha along the road then kill him', refers to the notion that as we find help and answers along the way, we must not elevate them to godlike status or remain attached to them, but must be prepared to let them go. In integrating the results of our hard work, it is important not to let the means become the ends.

> I meet so many people who are not moving on. One person can't meditate unless he's surrounded by particular crystals, mats or blankets. Another feels her world falls apart unless she sticks absolutely to her spiritual 'routine'. Another searches everywhere for sacred places to meditate because he can't find God in any other place.

Such an approach locks us into a fixed path and blocks out opportunities for continued deepening of our awareness and exploration of our potential. We may pass through phases where certain objects or practices are essential to where we are right then, but it is important to recognise when to move on and let go. Otherwise the object or the practice becomes an end in itself, a shadow trap that keeps us from bringing more of ourselves into the light.

Healers and carers may find that this happens with the various treatments and caring strategies used. The pills, the potions and the oils may become the only instruments we can use in our craft. And yet, the opportunities for healing may be much greater than this. What we do as healers undoubtedly impacts upon the recipients. Who we are may have an equal or even greater impact than what we do. Our being, the consciousness with which we approach each caring moment seems to be as potent in itself as any material or instrumental aspect of our work. Larry Dossey (1997) believes that there is an ever present danger in the field of complementary therapies, for example, where:

acupuncturists, herbal therapists and homeopaths … wield their therapies in a completely mechanical way. They have become so enchanted with the power of their 'device' that they have forgotten the non-local healing influences of empathy, love and compassion.

Perhaps those who have become attached to their healing or spiritual practices do so because it feels safer. The alternative is to explore and examine the possibilities of the therapeutic use of themselves, and to keep on doing so. Franz Kafka (1916) reminds us that 'sometimes it is safer to be in chains than to be free'. Breaking the comforting, secure chains that bind us takes courage.

2. SPIRITUAL FUNDAMENTALISM

Presenting itself to the world in the words of Pastor Niemoller, as darkness masking as light, we see the fundamentalist viewpoint almost everywhere. It is characterised by rigidity of thought, exclusion of all views beyond its own and, in the case of religion, literalist interpretation of scripture. Those who adopt such an approach find it difficult, if not impossible, to tolerate difference, and this intolerance may be demonstrated by individuals refusing to listen to any other view or participate in any practice other than their own. Worse, those who hold such views may seek to repress the words or deeds of those who disagree, finally seeking even to exterminate them. Such a worldview does not rest in the belief that it is right, but in the fear, however unconscious, that it is wrong. If there were true belief, there would be no fear, for faith removes fear. As it is, deep-seated fear – of difference, of openness, of inclusiveness – drives those who hold a fundamental viewpoint to seek to dominate all around them. Throughout history, we have see the worst effects of fundamentalism, when those who believe themselves to be absolutely right see nothing wrong in harming or disposing of those who disagree.

As soon as you look at the world through an ideology you are finished. No reality fits an ideology. Life is beyond that. That is why people are always searching for a meaning to life … Meaning is only found when you go beyond meaning. Life only makes sense when you perceive it as a mystery and it makes no sense to the conceptualising mind. (de Mello 1990)

These words by Anthony de Mello illustrate the difficulty facing those of a fundamentalist persuasion, in whatever belief system they operate: a world of uncertainty, difference, contradiction, questioning and mystery. A person who has not entered his own darkness to pass beyond fear will remain fearful, and being fearful, the only response may be to cling to one world-view. The alternative, a world of mystery and variety, is too terrifying to comprehend.

At a recent conference, we sought to include practices from many different faiths and therapies. Some odd views turned up. The aromatherapist questioned having an Alexander technique person present. The orthodox doctor was treated frostily

by some complementary therapists. A person describing herself as a Christian
objected to a workshop being run by a pagan or the use of incense in a ceremony.
A pagan didn't see the point of having a bishop present. And so it went on…

A fundamentalist view can creep into all arenas of thought, not just religion,
and be acted out in all manner of excluding ways. When we are rigid in our
beliefs, rooted in fear, the darkness is strengthened – in ourselves and in the
world around us.

3. SPIRITUAL TOURISM

In the early part of our thirst for self-discovery, we may find ourselves caught
up in endless searching in countless different places. Like a child in a toy shop,
there seems to be so much on offer that we want it all. A trick of the mind
seems to keep us moving from one thing to another, when we should be still.
We can travel anywhere, read, watch films of or participate in countless
approaches. We can open a magazine and find people selling us instant
healing, self-knowledge or enlightenment – try them out on Saturday, and if
they don't work have a go at a different one on Monday. While such freedom
of choice is one of the benefits of our ever-expanding universe, it can also
distract us with its endless possibility or promises of an easier option. It may
tempt us to give up on one when the going gets tough and the real hard work
has to be done. It is also worth noting that much choice:

does not necessarily contribute to spiritual freedom. The search for spirituality can
sometimes lead people to join spiritual groups that have all the characteristics of a
dysfunctional family; authoritarian parent figures that demand unquestioning
obedience and the abdication of responsibility for personal choices, as well as
various forms of addiction and co-dependency. (Vaughan 1995)

John Babbs (1991) writes:

I went last night, as I have so many other nights, to one of those wondrous New
Age gatherings. And I don't think I can take any more. I get sick. I must escape the
torture of being blessed to death during evenings such as this. There is something
frighteningly unreal about them that I can't quite put my finger on. All I know is
that afterwards I want to scream profanities, drink whiskey out of a bottle, go to
sleazy blues joints and chase wild, wild women. At this event a beautiful young
man told of his travels throughout the globe visiting sacred ceremonial sites – 400
all told. He has been around the world 14 times in his 34 years, living in many of
these places for months, sometimes years on end.

An episode of tourism may be beneficial, as we seek to find the right
approach for ourselves, be it a particular place, teacher or method. However,
there is likely to come a point when the touring has to stop and the hard
personal work is engaged in – it is simply not possible to bypass this labour
if we are to reach the light we seek.

I spent years travelling, literally inside myself and around the world. I read widely.
Went to ancient sacred sites. Took drugs. Sat at the feet of many great teachers

and some not so great. In the end, I began to awaken to a possibility that seemed so simple, so outrageously simple, that I couldn't believe it, and yet it continued to bubble up inside me, stronger each day. By chance, with Ram Dass, I told him of this, and I said 'After all this time I think I've found it, what I'm looking for, do you know where it is?' He nodded, and we both moved our hands simultaneously, pointed at our hearts, and said in perfect duet 'right here'. I went home, took up my meditation with renewed vigour and learned to find the teachers and teachings that were right under my nose all the time.

Very often what we need to illuminate the shadow is already with us. As suggested in Chapter 4, the spiritual discipline we may need may already be unnoticed around us in, for example a nearby teacher or group, the religion of our own particular culture, our work or our relationships. The Kabir (Bly 1990) summarises this poetically and beautifully:

> Are you looking for me? I am in the next seat.
> My shoulder is against yours.
> You will not find me in stupas, not in Indian shrine
> rooms, nor in synagogues, nor in cathedrals;
> not in masses, nor kirtans, not in legs winding
> around your neck, nor in eating nothing but vegetables.
> When you really look for me, you will find me instantly –
> you will find me in the tiniest house of time.
> Kabir says: Student, tell me, what is God?
> It is the breath inside the breath.

Easwaran's (1988) translation of the Upanishads gives an even more precise definition, stating:

'The Self, small as the thumb, dwelling in the heart, is like the sun shining in the sky … It may appear smaller than a hair's breadth, but know the self to be infinite'.

This notion, that what is within us is also beyond us, is replicated in many arenas of spiritual and mystical writing, and moves into much of the thinking of modern physics: the soul is in the body but the body is also in the soul; consciousness resides in the body but the body is also in consciousness.

4. SPIRITUAL ADDICTION

Another trap for the seeker awaits in the desire to repeat the 'highs'. The moments of clarity, revelation, understanding or bliss that come to those who live meditative, contemplative, reflective or prayerful life may become goals in themselves. Like an addiction, more and more enlightenment is pursued in order to keep getting the 'hit', but also, as with an addiction, it becomes more and more difficult, if not impossible, to repeat that first peak experience. Frances Vaughan (1995) notes how 'In order to continue the journey, the initiation experience, like all experiences, must be released'.

I had wonderful moments as things got clearer, and I found myself wanting more and more. I was impatient with people and the demands of ordinary life that kept me away from these. I took Ecstasy tablets, I was stunned by what I saw and felt, but found myself wanting to repeat the experience. The more I wanted it, the more it seemed to elude me. I also found myself hating the darkness that followed the light, blissful happy experience. I found myself wanting more and more to escape this darkness, of coming back into the ordinary world ... so I avoided people, worked more than ever with all my spiritual tools – prayer, meditation, Tarot reading – all of them seemed to be getting me nowhere. And I kept moving too, from one sacred or special site after another, one teacher, or class or therapy after another ... all chasing the same ends, which seemed even further out of reach the more I tried.

Caught up in the hunger for more beautiful experiences, we can end up working hard to avoid the dark; in so doing the blissful experiences too can evade us, and thereby the darker times can seem even darker. Without the grounding in everyday reality of all our experiences, both good and bad, we end up in endless pursuit of something that remains forever just out of reach. The way out of this trap is to let go of the meditative experiences, avoid judgments, stop longing for blissful episodes and accept whatever presents itself in life to be the teaching. The biblical story of a camel finding it easier to get through the eye of a needle than for a rich man to get to God is not just about material wealth. It also indicates that our possessions – which may be our attachments to things or to particular goals – are in themselves, the very hindrance that blocks us getting to where we want to be. Working with the dark has to be accepted as part of our overall work, and the darkness may be embodied in our wishes to avoid it. As Ram Dass (1997) says, 'Truth waits for eyes unclouded by longing'.

5. SPIRITUAL UNGROUNDING

Spiritual addiction and tourism are some of the ways that can keep us from moving on. They may have other impacts as well. There may seem to be little point in deepening our understanding and awareness, if we do not put this realisation to use in the world in some way. It is important to move beyond the pursuit of enlightenment for personal gratification only. The Upanishads ask the seeker to 'give', the Qur'an to 'be merciful', the Bible to be a good Samaritan. Buddhist texts include 'right action' as part of 'right living'. Others write of the need to be 'compassion in action' (Ram Dass & Bush 1992). David Steindl-Rast (1991) notes that:

Having discovered the Divine in the depths of his or her own soul, the adept must then find the Divine in all life. This is, in fact, the adept's principal obligation and responsibility. To put it differently, having drunk at the fountain of life, the adept must complete the spiritual opus and practice compassion on the basis of the recognition that everything participates in the universal field of the Divine.

Whether we adopt a theistic or atheistic stance, the message remains the same: deepen your understanding of yourself and your part in the scheme of things, but at some point, integrate the wanderings and the searchings, the therapies and the tools of the spiritual trade, and go out into the world and apply what you have learned. Retreating from the world in order to deepen our understanding of ourselves and our spiritual practice is an essential part of the process, but it does not mean that we have to remain in permanent retreat. Such an attachment to the safe haven away from the cares of the world becomes another form of spiritual materialism. We may need to spend time learning meditation with a local group, go into therapy or retreat to some remote Làmasery – whichever feels most right and appropriate for us. Such an escape, for a while, from ordinary reality, can help us to let go of everyday concerns and focus on the inner work we have to do, to pursue the inner pilgrimage for a while. Like all pilgrims, however, the journey should also lead us back into the world to bring what we have learned into action and integrate it into our daily lives.

Furthermore, this does not necessarily mean that we have to pack our bags, give up all our worldly possessions, and camp out with the homeless on the streets of London or head for the nearest trouble spot. The chances are that our opportunities for being compassionate in the world are already there, for instance, improving our relationships with our partners, friends, families or workmates, participating in local charitable work, or helping a distressed neighbour. All manner of ways present themselves to us every day. For those of us in caring situations, whether professionals such as doctors, nurses, social workers or other helpers, or whether as informal carers of loved ones, the openings to transform our work are countless. Bringing what we learn into our everyday lives continues the changing of the shadow into light.

6. SPIRITUAL GURUISM

The term 'guru' has been somewhat debased by common usage. We tend to apply it nowadays to anyone who seems to be an expert in his or her field and to whom we turn for that 'final word' of advice. In spiritual terms, a guru is different from a teacher. Ram Dass (1997) points out that 'The teacher points the way, the guru is the way'. Teachers, be they persons, events or things, all offer us opportunities for guidance and learning. A guru has already achieved that state of being, realisation and enlightenment that the seeker seeks – and such persons are few and far between. Mother Meera, Sai Baba, the Dalai Lama – these and others like them are often cited as modern-day gurus who have not sought to trap others as mindless servants.

However, the shadow lurks to capture the unwary. *The Cloud of Unknowing* (Wolters 1978) warns: 'It is quite possible for a young disciple, inexperienced and untested spiritually, to be deceived'. Anthony Storr (1996) lucidly portrays the effects of rampant egomania in certain individuals who use their insights to abuse and perhaps even destroy their followers. In studying such leaders as David Koresh, Jim Jones or Bhagwan Shree Rajneesh, we find a common thread running through their stories: an inflated belief in themselves and their single-minded view of the universe that leads both them and their followers ultimately along destructive paths.

> I was involved for quite a few years with a 'house church': a born-again Christian group with a very literal interpretation of the Bible. I went along with it for many years, even to the point of having my wife chosen for me. We had strict rules for behaviour, but I began to notice some inconsistencies. The leader told us all how to behave with our wives, but had an extramarital affair himself. He preached of the love of God, but told us people with AIDS were damned to hell.

It can be difficult to find a safe haven for guidance. However, there are some points worth considering as warning signs when checking out the suitability of a person as a spiritual teacher or guide:

- Does the teacher seek to draw you into their sphere of influence and hold you there, or do they act as planet to a satellite on a space journey? That is, when you come close to them, do they seek to empower you to move on to complete your journey, even if it means leaving them behind? Teachers who need devotees to act out their own needs for power or deal with their own inadequacies are not really going to help you.

- Does he pass the Deikman (1990) test of spiritual advancement? It has one main question: how does he get along with his wife? In other words, what are his relationships like? How does he treat you and others around him. In other words, does he practice what is preached when he talks of peace, love, understanding and positive relationships. Does he 'walk his talk'? Larry LeShan (1974) says: 'If these relationships are not of the kind you admire, then it really doesn't matter how steadily he looks at you behind his steel grey eyes, how silently he sits in a perfect lotus position, or how impressive he looks in robe and beard. Cross him off your list and look elsewhere'.

- Do they ask you to trust them completely, as it will take you years to become enlightened, so do as they say without question? It is important to accept things not because they come from a great teacher, but because they feel *absolutely right to you*. A good teacher will ask you to trust your own intuition and judgement, not to abandon them. Your own critical faculties are tools to serve you on your quest.

- Do they demand that you accept their authority and theirs alone, suppressing your own will completely? If so, move on and find another.

- Do they promise you what you need, but tell you that the doctrines are exclusive and secret and cannot be revealed to the uninitiated (As LeShan[1995] notes, 'Can you imagine a Socrates, a Jesus or a Buddha telling that his wisdom was to be kept secret?').

- Do they promise what you need, but first of all you must give up to them, for example, your money, your possessions, your relationships, your job or your body?

- Does the teacher expect you to look up to them uncritically at all times?

- Is the teacher running an organisation that amounts to little more than a big business?

- Does the teacher (and the same here applies to many New Age health 'gurus') or those who follow them tend towards 'spiritual blaming'? This is an attitude which suggests that your inability to get enlightened/understand/ cure your illness is your own fault because, for example: you are not evolved enough; you are too stupid; you do not work hard enough; you have not given enough; you have not resolved childhood issues around your mother; its your karma to be sick; or you have not cleared out a past life.
- Is the teacher or belief system packed with oppressive groups who use peer pressure to make you conform to their point of view? Repressive groups tend to deal with problems by denial and avoidance rather than by generating faith and trust. Jones (1996) notes how in such groups, 'Devotees are often told simply to forget their problems, get involved in some project, work harder, believe or have a baby'. Pathological groups like this need to be avoided.

If you cannot get clear answers to questions like these, and suspect that you may be controlled rather than empowered by a particular teacher, then it is best to 'seek the nearest exit immediately!' (LeShan 1995). A teacher or guru who tells us what do all the time undermines our ability to make decisions for ourselves, and to fully participate in the work that has to be done. However, with these reservations in mind, this does not mean that we should shun working with a teacher or guru completely. Indeed, working with our darkness with the help of a trusted guide or adviser, or a group of them, has many benefits. Perhaps working with several rather than one provides a wider breadth of teaching and an insurance policy against falling into guruism. The teacher–seeker relationship should be one which fosters growth in our own awareness and abilities, and then seeks to let us go when the work that can be done with them is completed. Perhaps it is sometimes better to learn from many rather than one to avoid the pitfalls, and to rigorously appraise what is on offer using the 10 statements above as a starting point. Our teachers and spiritual directors may take many forms when we look to another person: priest or therapist, healer or counsellor, or, that rare find, a true guru who *is* the way. They can be there as friends and guides when we are unclear about the meaning of our experiences. When we become confused or dispirited, they can clarify things and encourage us on our way. The true teacher emerges as companion along the way, journeying with you while they are needed, then letting you go onward when your journey takes a different route from themselves. Teachers or gurus are indeed masters, but first and foremost, they are masters of themselves and their craft – not of us.

7. SPIRITUAL APARTHEID

In seeking after the sacred, there can be a tendency to separate spiritual practice from other things, and it thereby becomes something we do on certain occasions or at a particular ceremony. Being open and loving can become something we reserve for some people and not for others.

I found it easy being in the retreat to feel open, to feel connected to others in a loving way. I noticed I was patient and accepting, just letting other people do their stuff without much judging or criticising. When I get back home, it's the same old thing. I find myself behaving in just the same way as before, it seems the only way to get on in the world and do the things I have to do. So I end up with two lives at work in me. One is the ordinary, the everyday, where I seem to be the same as I always was; the other is those moments – perhaps an occasional weekend or a week away in meditation somewhere. It's fine while I'm there, everything is loving and beautiful, then its – Bang! – back into the other stuff like nothing had changed. It was just the same with my mother and father, I remember. They'd be beasts to be with all week, but then Sunday was church and everything would be sweet and holy for a few hours, then back to 'normal' the next day.

Apartheid was built on the notion that some people are superior to others. Thus, a close cousin of spiritual apartheid is spiritual snobbery, evidenced by those who tell us repeatedly that they have either suffered more than us or are more advanced, enlightened or spiritually sophisticated than us. People who are participating in expanding their consciousness do not have to tell you that; it is obvious by their actions. They know that 'more' or 'less' are very relative terms and are largely irrelevant to spirituality. We are all enlightened; we have only to become conscious of it.

The 'holier than thou' attitude, rooted in fear that needs a sense of superiority to neutralise it, is a common phenomenon among seekers of the sacred. As the sacred takes us ever more into understanding the unity that underlies everything, the individualist ego reacts to what might seem a frightening possibility: that underlying our individuality is the reality that we are all the same and part of the same. Interconnectedness is an awesome concept, and we may respond to its enormity with fear, by discounting it. Separation of the self from the 'common run' of others, either through a sense of superiority or separating the sacred altogether, is another trick of the shadow that keeps us from entering the 'all that is'.

In a world of many demands, threats and fears it can seem almost impossible to see the sacred all around us, and to be who we really are in the face of seemingly impossible odds stacked against us. And yet, as Gretel Ehrlich (cited in Sullivan 1987), poet and novelist writes: 'Sacred or secular, what is the difference? If every atom inside our bodies was once a star, then it is all sacred and all secular at the same time'. This notion that 'all is one' is a repeated theme in almost every ancient and modern sacred text, and it is now mirrored in the field of quantum physics. The Persian mystic, Abu Hamid Muhammad Al-Ghazzali (cited in McLuhan 1996) takes up this view: 'Stones, plants, animals, the earth, the sky, the stars, the elements, in fact everything in the universe reveals to us the knowledge, power and will of its creator'. The Upanishads (Easwaran 1988) echo this in the line: 'This entire cosmos, whatever is still or moving, is pervaded by the Divine'.

Separating secular and sacred can lead us into the shadow of 'being good in this situation, but not being good in another'. We become confusing and inconsistent in our approach. Speaking of the 'Father' in the Gospel of

St Thomas, Jesus said 'It is I who am the all. From me did all come forth, and unto me did the all extend. Split a piece of wood, and I am there. Lift up the stone, and you will find me there' (Koester & Lambdin 1996).

If everything is interconnected, as ancient scripture and modern physics suggest, then simple spacial contact of things is only a small part of the grander scheme of connection. We reduce our view of the world and its potential for us when we separate the sacred from 'the rest'. Every moment offers opportunities to become more awakened; every moment is a continuing unfolding of the universe. To see it otherwise runs the risk that our spiritual 'side' is relegated to particular events, rituals or persons. Everything is spiritual, everything is sacred, whether at the extremes of darkness or light, the same presence runs throughout it. Our challenge is to become aware of and find the right relationship with it. To seek to see the world only in a blissed-out state of mind is as much an illusion as to see it as only a place of terrible shadow: it is both, and neither, and we can work with these teaching as a whole if we are to bring transformation into the world in whatever way is right for us.

LOVING THE DARK

In this chapter we have sought to suggest that an exploration of the shadow side of ourselves is a vital part of our own healing, of entering into right relationship with ourselves and perhaps our God. This in turn allows us to be in right relationship with others as we reach out to care and heal. We cannot avoid the darkness, although we may often try (Figure 5.2). Frances Vaughan (1995) suggests that 'If freedom is the goal, the seeker needs to recognise how it can be subverted in the name of progress toward any unattainable ideal, such as never having negative emotions'. If the negative is unavoidable, then the solution seems to be to accept it as something to work with, as a teacher, no matter how difficult it may be to face it. The great Irish poet, W B Yeats (Webb 1991) echoes this in the poem 'Ribh Considers Christian Love Insufficient' with the following lines:

> Why should I seek for love or study it?
> It is of God and passes human wit;
> I study hatred with great diligence,
> For that's a passion in my own control,
> A sort of besom that can clear the soul
> Of everything that is not mind or sense.
>
> Why do I hate man, woman or event?
> That is a light my jealous heart has sent.
> From terror and deception freed it can
> Discover impurities, can show at last
> How soul may walk when all such things are past,
> How soul walked before such things began.

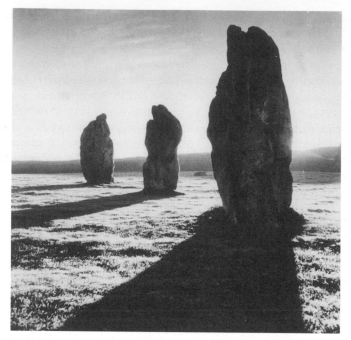

Figure 5.2 Standing stones: the sacred is found both in shadow and light. © Laurence Winram, reprinted with permission.

For some, working with the darkness may be a terrifying ordeal. Confronting the wounds of the past – bereavement, pain, injustice done to us or the fear of death (as Mark Mattoussek [1996] illustrates in his life with HIV) – is the stuff of enlightenment. But, as Jung (1959) reiterated, 'We do not become enlightened by imagining figures of light, but by making the darkness conscious'. This whole chapter has been based on this belief.

Modern western culture, in particular, has become very goal orientated. This applies no less to those who begin the search for the sacred and, as we have suggested, this includes an exploration of the shadow. However, the idea of a defined end may be an illusion too. The search for the sacred has no endpoint, but is an ongoing process.

When I became aware of my exploration over 20 years ago, I thought some day there would be a finish to it. I'm not so sure about that now. Maybe there is no end to it, maybe it's just participating in the endless creation and unfolding of the cosmos, I don't know. I do know that I don't mind not knowing, that I am comfortable with the mystery and the uncertainty. I do know that things I once thought to be clear and sorted out, return from time to time to be re-explored, to be revisited, and with each of these, even now, I still find new insights, new lessons to be learned.

This notion of an endless journey, process rather than outcome, can seem daunting, if not overwhelming, but consciousness is boundless, and there are no limits to the dimensions of consciousness to be explored, even though we may end up returning to the same point when all our wanderings are done. Cavafy's poem, 'Ithaka' (1995) expands on this theme, reminding us not to 'hurry the journey at all, better it lasts for years, so you are wealthy with all you have gained along the way'.

The idea of the journey or pilgrimage is repeated again and again in many spiritual writings, from the exploration of the 'interior castle' of St Theresa or the pilgrim's progress of Bunyan. Pilgrims are 'persons in motion – passing through territories not their own – seeking something we might call completion, or perhaps the word clarity will do as well, a goal to which only the spirit's compass points the way ... even though we may not give ourselves the name. Words and their meanings are animated by currents of energy ... summoning us to be on our way' (Niehbuhr 1984). Countless possibilities may prompt the summons, from a life crisis to a moment of quiet reflection. Whether we follow or not is our choice, but, perhaps eventually, to follow is the only choice there is.

The negative, the shadow, is our teaching too; it is the grist for the mill. To avoid it is to lock ourselves into a kind of spiritual bondage that must ultimately demand release. Perhaps the only thing to fear is fear itself, for when the light shines in the dark, the dark dissipates and its power is lost, and perhaps we become more interesting and joyful people to be around in the process. It is our experience, indeed, that some of the most open, loving, fascinating and 'whole' people we have had the pleasure of meeting have themselves had the courage to move through (not around) the dark night of the soul. They have lived through histories of terrible wounds from which they have been healed by turning dark into light. But then, are we not all wounded healers? Love the darkness:

You darkness, that I come from,
I love you more than all the fires
that fence the world,
for the fire makes
a circle of light for everyone,
and then no one outside learns of you.
but the darkness pulls in everything;
shapes and fires, animals and myself,
how easily it gathers them!—
powers and people—

and it is possible a great energy
is moving near me.

I have faith in nights.

Rainer Maria Rilke (1981)

REFERENCES

Attar F ud-din 1984 Darbandi A, Davis D (trans) The conference of the birds. Penguin, London
Babbs J 1991 New age fundamentalism. In: Zwieg C, Abrams J (eds) 1991 Meeting the shadow – the hidden power of the dark side of human nature. Putnam, New York
Barasch M 1993 The healing path. Arkana/Penguin, London
Bly R (trans) 1990 The Kabir. Book 44 of the ecstatic poems of Kabir. Harper Row, London
Bly R 1991 The long bag we drag behind us. In: Zwieg C, Abrams J (eds) 1991 Meeting the shadow – the hidden power of the dark side of human nature. Putnam, New York
Cavafy C P 1995 Keeley E (trans) The essential Cavafy. Ecco, Hopewell
Coelho P 1993 The alchemist. Harper Collins, London
Deikman A 1990 The wrong way home; uncovering the patterns of cult behaviour in American society. Beacon, Boston
de Mello A 1990 Awareness. Doubleday, New York
Dossey L 1997 The forces of healing. Alternative Therapies in Health and Medicine 3(5): 8–14
Easwaran E (trans) 1988 The Upanishads. Arkana, London
Flanagan S 1989 Hildegard of Bingen – a visionary life. Routledge, London
Gibran K 1933 The garden of the prophet. Harmondsworth, Penguin
Hample S, Marshall E 1975 Children's letters to God. Fount, Hammersmith
Harvey A 1991 Hidden journey. Rider, London
Hillman J 1996 The soul's code. Warner, New York
Jones J 1996 In the middle of this road we call our life. Harper Collins, London
Jung C G 1959 Symbols of transformation. Bollinger, Princeton
Kafka F 1916 (reprinted 1974) Metamorphosis. Penguin, Harmondsworth
Koester H, Lambdin T O 1996 The gospel of Thomas. In: Robinson J M (ed) The Nag Hammadi library in English. Brill, Leiden
LeShan L 1974 How to meditate. Harper Collins, London
LeShan L 1995 Mobilising the life force, treating the individual. Alternative Therapies in Medicine 1(1): 63–69
Mattoussek M 1996 Sex, death and enlightenment. Riverhead Books, New York
McLuhan T C 1996 Cathedrals of the spirit. Thorsons, London
Niebuhr R R 1984 Pilgrims and pioneers. Parabola 9(3): 7
Ram Dass, Bush M 1992 Compassion in action. Bell, New York
Ram Dass 1997 The Book of Grace. Hanuman Foundation Tape Library, San Anselmo
Rilke R 1981 Bly R (trans) Selected poems of Rainer Maria Rilke. Harper & Row, London
Robinson J (ed) 1988 The Nag Hammadi library. Harper & Row, San Francisco
Rumi 1994 Moyne J, Barks C (trans) Say I am you. Maypop, Athens
St John of the Cross 1973 Zimmerman B (trans) The dark night of the soul. Clarke, Cambridge
Steindl-Rast D 1991 The shadow in Christianity. In: Zwieg C, Abrams J (eds) Meeting the shadow – the hidden power of the dark side of human nature. Putnam, New York
St Theresa of Avila 1995 Van de Weyer R (trans) The interior castle. Harper Collins, London
Storr A 1996 Feet of clay – a study of gurus. Harper Collins, London
Sullivan C (ed) 1987 The legacy of light. Knopf, New York
Thich Nhat Hanh 1993 taken from: please call me by my true names. In: Present moment; wonderful moment. Rider, London
Underhill E 1911 Mysticism. Methuen, London
Vaughan F 1995 Shadows of the sacred. Quest, Wheaton
Watson L 1980 Lifetide. Bantam, London
Webb T (ed) 1991 W B Yeats selected poetry. Penguin, Harmondsworth
Wolters C (trans) 1978 The cloud of unknowing. Penguin, London
Wilber K 1991 Taking responsibility for your shadow. In: Zwieg C, Abrams J (eds) Meeting the shadow – the hidden power of the dark side of human nature. Putnam, New York
Zweig C, Abrams J (eds) 1991 Meeting the shadow – the hidden power of the dark side of human nature. Putnam, New York

Epilogue

We are not human beings having a spiritual experience, but
spiritual beings having a human experience.

Jean Shinoda Bolen

Our real journey in life is interior; it is a matter of growth,
deepening, and of an ever greater surrender to the creative action of
love and grace in our hearts. Never was it more necessary for us to
respond to that action.

Thomas Merton

We have sought to bring attention to the spiritual malaise in many caring
relationships, and from the evidence we have cited, the malaise cannot only
be confirmed, but its depth and severity are clear. Its effects are profound.
Some people, a minority according to the surveys we have cited, appear to
be comfortable in the maelstrom of modern healthcare. This may be because
they have walled themselves off from the madness to keep themselves safe
(but in so doing lose the possibility of connection with others) or they have
attained that place in themselves where they can feel whole and centred. In
this state of being, they are able to work in the world compassionately, without
harm to themselves and others. Such a state is not possible without a spiritual
exploration of our roots and our connectedness to all that is.

Sri Aurobindo (1970) characterised spirituality as:

... not a high intellectuality, not idealism, not an ethical turn of mind or moral purity
or austerity, not religiosity or an ardent and exalted emotional fervour, not even a
compound of all these excellent things; a mental belief, creed or faith, an emotional
aspiration, a regulation of conduct according to religious or ethical formula are not
spiritual achievement and experience. Spirituality is in its essence, an awakening to
the inner reality of our being, to a spirit, self, soul which is other than our mind, life
and body, an inner aspiration to know, to feel, to be that, to enter into contact with
the greater reality beyond and pervading the universe which inhabits also our own
being.

Our pursuit of our (the) spirituality is essential if we are to become
grounded in right relationship with ourselves and others in the world. This
sacred act, followed by millions down the ages, is true holism; coming home
to the reality that we are not separate, that we do not have to be 'in charge'.
Grounded in this inner sacred space, we can be readily available to birth the
sacred into the rest of the world, or at least what we see as our part of it.
Grounded in inner and outer sacred space, we can work without burnout and
self-destruction.

We have contended that much of the sickness and burnout in caring
relationships has its source in issues beyond resources and conditions of

work. Indeed where these fail us, we suggest that they are the products of a failure in right relationship throughout the healthcare system and society as a whole. So many attempts to right the wrongs, from improving pay and conditions to changing whole systems (be they healthcare or social and political systems) seem to flounder. One system replaces another, yet the flaws continue under another guise. We hunger for that right place to be, endlessly changing jobs, roles or partners in our search, and dulling the pain of the struggle with sex, drugs or drink. Many are damaged by this hunger. Some seem to sense the source of the restlessness.

 The search begins with a restless feeling, as if one were being watched. One turns in all directions and sees nothing. Yet one senses that there is a source for this deep restlessness; and the path that leads there is not a path to a strange place, but the path home. ('But you are home' cries the Witch of the North. 'All you have to do is wake up!') (Jones 1996).

Struggle and suffering are grace – they are wake-up calls for the divine, to our destiny, they provide us with the darkness that can be transmuted to light; they are our teachers on the way.

If the path home, to right relationship with the self and beyond is the key, we can but wonder how the world would be transformed if even a small proportion of all the carers responded to that restlessness and began the

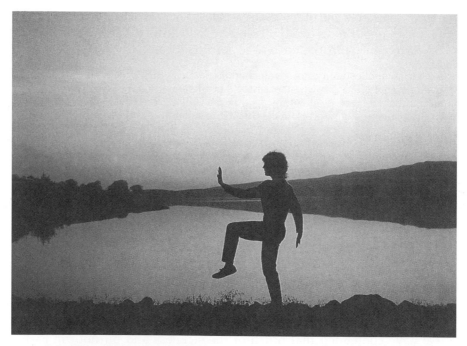

Figure E. 1 Being still, for even a moment, may awaken us to the sacred within and without.
© Forder & Forder, reprinted with permission.

journey. A journey that is not a self-congratulatory passage inward, a retreat from one reality into another, but a cycle of enlightenment. Deepening our understanding of ourselves and our sacred source, we turn back to bring that into the world and change it, not just by doing, but by being different. Our enlightenment affects all around us. The spiritual journey we advocate is an action spirituality. The search for the sacred is not a retreat from the world, an escape from, or complacency toward suffering, but a shift of consciousness that empowers us to participate in the creation of new realities. Come home to yourself, and having found home, be available to consciously aid in the coming home, the healing of others. The sacred, enlightenment, consciousness are not ends in themselves, indeed they cannot be sought like the source of a river. They are present, right here, right now. All we have to do is wake up to that (Figure E. 1). Right relationship begins and ends with ourselves. John Main, a Benedictine monk (cited in McLuhan 1996) states that 'The Kingdom is not a place we are going, but rather an experience we carry with us on every breath'.

In seeking to redress the ills of the caring system, we have therefore focused on relationships, and suggested many paths to follow. We have also suggested that this process is not without risk. However, we have noted ways in which it can be done safely. The alternative is the status quo with all the damage it is currently doing, and that to us is not an alternative.

Finding the right teacher(s), taking care of ourselves and being alert to the signs of charlatans and quackery are part of the safety net. Organisations, teams and individuals can do much to develop right relationship locally. We can recognise the signs and symptoms of stress for what they are, not just the product of overworking but also over-giving, and create environments where such signs are respected and acted upon. We can recognise that, at a deeper level, a burning out carer is having not just a psychological and physical crisis, but a spiritual one as well. A spiritual emergency can be a time of great danger; its presentation, especially in western cultures is almost invariably branded with some form of psychiatric label. The resulting 'treatment' tends only to repress the symptoms, rather than create a safe space in which they can be explored and worked through. The dividing line between madness and mysticism is very fine; as Joseph Campbell (1988) observed, 'the madman is drowning in the same water in which the mystic swims with delight'. A psychological emergency may therefore often be a spiritual emergency, an existential crisis in which old norms of meaning, values and purpose have broken down and body, mind and soul struggle to stay on an even keel. Such a crisis is also an opportunity, if we would but recognise it, for a spiritual emergency presents us with the gateway for a spiritual emergence.

At the Sacred Space Foundation, we have been exploring ways of helping carers who reach such a crisis. Many who call us for help are clearly suffering great anguish and stress brought on by working conditions and the costs of caring relationships. It says a great deal about carers that they very often have avoided reporting their distress to the employers or organisations that are supposed to support them. They feel unable to indicate to the wider world that they are not coping in some way. A suggestion of seeking conventional help, e.g. in the form of a sedative or antidepressant from a GP, is generally treated with horror. In part, they feel unable to tell anyone of their difficulties, not least their own doctor, but there is also a common response to the thought of resorting to drugs, which are seen as a sign of weakness. Such superhood views belie the fact that the person has probably been taking addictive 'drugs' in other forms already to dampen the strain – smoking, drinking, sex, shopping – whatever it takes to distract the mind from the unfolding struggle. There is nothing intrinsically wrong in using the available help, even conventional drugs, to get us safely stabilised in a crisis. The issues of concern, as we have suggested, are why we feel so guilt-ridden or fearful in doing so, and how we can use them as a vehicle to prepare us to move onward by doing the deeper work that is needed, and not as a prop to shore up the status quo and keep the darkness at bay.

Moving out of the spiritual emergency requires complex inner work and attentive, creative, expert support. We have found the following pattern to be helpful in dealing with and preventing a crisis, and keeping us going along our path:

- Access to sanctuary: a quiet, safe place of retreat, where the person can be as quiet and alone as they wish, or can work with others. Stepping out of the everyday world for a little while into a safe haven allows an opportunity for reflection and re-energising.
- Working with techniques for insight. exploring dreams, reflective practice, career counselling, psychotherapy, prayer, meditation, labyrinth walking and so on, as we suggested in Chapter 4, with the support of a teacher, guide or therapist.
- Caring for the body: an exercise programme within the person's capabilities, from gentle walks to mountain climbing, the provision of good food, and perhaps someone to prepare it for you.
- Outreach and networking: access to help when the person leaves sanctuary, knowing that a contact point for guidance and further support remains. There is no final 'discharge', because difficulties and challenges are part of life, but people need to know the sources of help that are available, within themselves, at the retreat and from others in their daily lives. Networking and meeting with groups of others who are also seekers, and with whom we can share experiences and from whom we can derive support is invaluable.
- Aftercare programmes: individuals need to work out a plan of action for their return to the wider world, how they will resolve outstanding problems, attend to their whole wellbeing, work in relationships differently and so on. This may involve anything from an agreed approach to employers to a change of diet, from plans to create new relationships in the caring context to

maintaining a daily meditation. Finding alternatives that meet our needs are helpful as is building them into a regular routine that is realistic. As we suggested in Chapters 3 and 4, each person needs to commit themselves to an ongoing programme of personal and spiritual development, so that the emergency does not recur, better still is prevented and, more importantly, we achieve that shift of consciousness where sanctuary, the safe sacred space of being centred and whole, remains with us always

At the Sacred Space Foundation, one of our primary concerns is not just to deal with the crisis, but to hold the space, the sacred space, in which people can repair, refresh and renew themselves. More is needed. It is necessary to work with people so that they do not become addicted to retreat instead of finding right relationship and ways to live in the world around them. It may be necessary to work with employers and caring organisations to change the culture of non-caring and develop right relationship there; also to work with teams and other carers to develop right relationship in these arenas. It is also necessary for individuals to find and remain in right relationship with themselves.

Moving beyond retreat is important, getting past the idea that the person is 'going back' to their usual way of life. Without this, the crisis will simply return in one form or another. When we learn to take care of ourselves, set limits and boundaries, find practices that nourish and develop us as whole persons, then we can come home to that place in ourselves which is every place. Sacred space can be something that transcends the narrow view of a house or a sanctuary that we can go to when times get bad. We all may need a retreat of some sort from time to time, but this can become just another 'drug' to dull the senses if it is something we do only in crisis, in the difficult times, to put stress at bay for a little while. We thus have some reservations about the countless health farms, rest and recuperation centres that have been set up in recent years. If all we do is retire from the world for a little while, eat and exercise well and then go back into the same world that we left, then very little is accomplished save a short respite from the anguish of our caring relationships. All we are doing in these circumstances is fire fighting.

More structured and deliberate work is needed to free us from this pattern where we lurch from crisis to comforter and back again. A concerted effort is needed to bring change not just to those in crisis, but into our everyday lives – for ourselves, those we care for and those we work with and for. By pursuing our journey along the lines we have suggested, we follow what Carlos Castaneda (1968) in *The Teachings of Don Juan* and Jack Kornfield (1993) at the Spirit Rock Centre (a Buddhist-based centre of meditation and spiritual nurturance in the USA) have called a 'path with heart'. The path of the heart is that which has meaning, nurturance and purpose for us. Action and intent that feel absolutely right for us and our place in the world. The many paths we have described in Chapters 3 and 4 are heart paths. All of them are paths of love – toward the self and others and all that is. As Frances Vaughan (1995) writes that love 'which transcends reason' is an 'all pervasive, essential quality of existence, a creative resource of inexhaustible abundance. It seems that the further we go on the spiritual path, the more we become aware of love's presence in our lives'.

As paths of love, all the strategies we have suggested differ from much of what is currently on offer to those in the mainstream of caring, to change organisations, cultures and relationships. Too much emphasis is placed on power and control, on changing systems and reorganising structures and hierarchies. Our approach indicates that such short-term, reactionary measures tend to simply shift the power and structures around, giving an impression of change, but in reality changing very little. The chess pieces are moved around the board, but the game remains the same, the order unchanged, the regrouping constant. There are many paths of the heart; all draw on the power of love and trust, not of fear and control. If the third millennium is to be spiritual, then the 'new order' can only emerge using the energy of spirit – and that is love.

In pursuing the paths of the heart, we can also escape the trap of moving from one set of crutches to another to get us through life. Meditation, retreat, work on relationships, the path of service, labyrinth walking – these and all the other techniques we have touched upon can feed and strengthen our souls and move us beyond notions of 'going back'. When we have so attended to the nurturance of our spirit that we have truly come home, we can let go of whatever methods we have chosen. Resting easy in ourselves, there is no longer any 'going back' or 'going to'. Having awakened to the sacred space within ourselves and fallen into right relationship with it, we awaken also to the sacred that is in all things, the potential of right relationship with all things. No 'going back', just here, now, always. Right relationship is being fully present in the moment. 'Be here, now' as Ram Dass (1978) says.

ROOM FOR OPTIMISM

The picture that emerges from our exploration of the evidence of stress and burnout among carers seems bleak. Yet, if there is dark and light in everything, it needs to be noted that awareness of the difficulties of so many carers is prompting action – by individuals themselves, by organisations and by governments. The tendency to blame the victim, or for organisations to look for quick-fix structural changes, is not universally shared. Many groups are demonstrating ethical and spiritual approaches to business practices as we have shown, and some enlightened healthcare organisations are following suit. Individuals in all corners of society are working away to effect change.

More people are 'waking up', and it may be that more people are waking up at this time than ever before. At times when a special date is looming, there is a tendency to see the possibility of major shifts in world history occurring.

With the millennium at cusp as we write (a date of great significance to many, but by no means all, of the world's population), it may be that there is a discernible shift in the air. Some in the so-called New Age movement see this as a paradigm shift, a time of great change in consciousness as humanity takes on a new world-view that embraces compassion for all of creation and pushes onward with a resurgent spirituality. Anyone caught up in one of the world's families, watching the rain forests burn, witnessing the handiwork of yet another brutal despot, hearing the thundering of the literalists and fundamentalists, noticing yet another of the planet's precious life forms slip quietly into extinction, or any number of other catastrophes we could cite of environmental and social degradation – such a person might indeed have grounds for seeming a little more cynical.

While bigotry and fundamentalism seem to rise inexorably, we also see huge numbers of people pursuing their personal spiritual paths without hierarchical bodies or dogma to control them. In the macho world of politics and business, there is at the same time a renewal of the spirit of community responsibility and ethical practices. As the powerful multinationals flourish, local community action groups and trading partnerships expand. Environmental degradation is counterbalanced by rising ecopraxis and action groups to halt and reverse it. The old power games in healthcare are shifting and, for example, the time-worn rituals of (male) dominant doctor and (female) subservient nurse or patient are slipping away. The thrust towards patient empowerment continues apace, and there are signs of the professionals realigning, developing new models of professionalism which do not rely upon elitist dominance of knowledge and practice and an obedient laity, but focusing on concepts of partnership, power sharing and cooperation. The barriers to different forms of healthcare practice are slowly crumbling as integration of services and practices is deemed ever more desirable.

All this goes on, of course, at the same time as the old models and approaches are perpetuated. If the old paradigm, the masculine, Piscean world of structures, order, power, control rooted in fear of freedom is indeed passing into the feminine, Aquarian age of flattened hierarchies, decentralised power, personal and spiritual liberation, then it is unlikely to be a sudden ending of one and start of the new. The two will exist side by side for many years to come, if not forever. We do not know. Indeed, we tend toward the view that it is not a case of either/or, either masculine or feminine, scientific or intuitive, reason or feelings, but an integration, a harmonising of both forces in an individual and collective spirituality that would be a truly transformative paradigm shift for the world. To achieve this goal, one of the central tenets of this book has been to encourage the personal, spiritual search of right relationship – of the sacred that is in us and in all things. Each person can choose the path of the heart, and for each it will be unique, but the endpoint will be the same.

It needs to be remembered, however, that the notion of a personal search is not accepted everywhere. Some or parts of the established religions frown upon anything that might challenge dogma, credal or Episcopalian authority. They argue that a personal spiritual search is too dangerous without the safety of the orthodox container. More and more people seem to be demonstrating, as we suggested in Chapter 3, that this approach no longer obtains. How the religious bodies will respond to this burgeoning individual approach to spirituality may determine their own futures as much as the seekers' futures. The attempt by some to reign in 'heresy' and hold the dogmatic line seems to be having a counterproductive effect. Artress (1995) and theologians like her suggest that a new accommodation of the personal and collective spiritual journey will have to be reached by the established religions.

At a conference in Durham in 1997 on the theme of spirituality and health, an evening debate was held about the proper role of the carer in relation to spirituality. Close to tears, one delegate said that she found it difficult to consider the spirituality of others in an organisation where she felt so neglected herself. Going to work had become a source of stress and pain, instead of joy and fulfilment. It was a place of non-connection in relationships. It was a place where healing had been sacrificed on the altar of cost-effectiveness. 'How can I go back to work', she asked 'when my heart and soul are not welcome there?'

Bringing the heart and soul into caring relationships, be they at home or work, is achievable. It is not an impossible dream. Organisations, teams and individuals can actively transform the context of care into a sacred space (Plate 10). We can do so by creating 'caring for the carers' approaches at all levels. We can do so by examining and adjusting the resources and systems that support caring relationships. We can do so most powerfully by attending to our own spiritual path, being in the world in ways which nourish and support ourselves and others. Although we have focused in this book on carers, both lay and professional, in the field of healthcare, we suspect that the principles we have discussed are generalisable to all relationships at work or home. Right relationship in the spheres we have suggested underpins all the ways we are in the world.

And the end of all this journeying? It is to arrive at a great truth, that the sacred has never been far away. Mother Meera (1991) reminds us that everything is available to us; we just have to ask for it. What our heart has sought was not a distant goal to be pursued across the globe in ashrams or monasteries or the tops of mountains or deep in the ocean. It was, is, right here, right now – we just had to wake up to it, to nudge our consciousness into seeing the world and ourselves as the sacred space we have always been. In changing our consciousness, we can change our actions This is the real, loving power available to transform that which is around us to be the same as that which is within us. Right relationship within and without, evolving to the point where there is no in or out, just here, now.

We cannot heal others, we can only care for and about them. This caring is acted out in the things we do to heal, in the treatments we prescribe and perform, in the environments we create which seek to rest the recipient of care in a loving, nurturing ambience. People can only heal themselves. Over and above anything we say or do to heal another or relieve their suffering, is who and how we are. We can witness caring and healing emerge as we become who we are, our true sacred selves. The work we do on right relationship is the means to that end, the passageway that allows the heart and soul to emerge in caring relationships and all that surrounds them. Sacred space is the place of healing. As it flashes into our awareness, our consciousness, we see that it was obvious. How could we have missed it? How could we have passed it by? There, right under our noses, all the time! Sacred space? It is our Selves.

REFERENCES

Artress L 1995 Walking a sacred path. Riverhead, New York
Campbell J 1988 The power of myth. Doubleday, New York
Castaneda C 1968 The teachings of don Juan – a Yaqui way of knowledge. Arkana, London
Jones J 1996 In the midst of this path we call our life. HarperCollins, London
Kornfield J 1993 A path with heart. Bantam, London
McLuhan T C 1996 Cathedrals of the spirit. Thorsons, London
Mother Meera 1991 Answers. Rider, London
Ram Dass 1978 Be here now. Crown, New York
Sri Aurobindo 1970 The life divine. Sri Aurobindo Ashram, Pondicherry
Vaughan F 1995 Shadows of the sacred. Quest, Wheaton

Useful addresses

Bristol Cancer Help Centre
Grove House
Cornwallis Grove
Clifton
Bristol BS8 4PG
UK

British Association of Therapeutic Touch (BATT)
Highland Hall
Renwick
Penrith
Cumbria CA10 1JL
UK

Commonweal
Box 316
Bolinas
CA 94924
USA

The Findhorn Foundation
The Park
Forres IV36 3TZ
UK

Gesundheidt Institute
HC64 Box 167
Hillsborough,
West Virginia 24946
USA

Glasgow Homeopathic Hospital
1000 Great Western Road
Glasgow GL12 0NR
UK

Global Network Spiritual Success
PO Box 1001
Del Mar
CA 92014
USA

Greenleaf Servant Leader Network
All Saints Road
Sutton
Surrey SM1 3DA
UK

The Hart Centre
2 Harts Gardens
Guildford
Surrey GU2 6QA
UK

Institute for Human Development
Burnts House
Chelwood
Bristol BS18 4NL
UK

Mother Meera
Oberdorf 4a
65599 Dornburg-Thalheim
Germany

National Association for Staff Support (NASS)
9 Caradon Close
Woking
Surrey GU21 3DU
UK

Planetree Health Resource Center
2040 Webster Street
San Francisco
CA 94115
USA

Sacred Space Foundation
Highland Hall
Renwick
Penrith
Cumbria CA10 1JL
UK

SEVA Foundation
108 Spring Lake Drive
Chelsea
MI 48118
USA

Social Venture Network Europe
PO Box 937
1000AX
Amsterdam
Holland

Spirit Rock Centre
PO Box 909
Woodacre
CA 94973
USA

Veriditas
World Wide Labyrinth Project
Grace Cathedral
1100 California Street
San Francisco 94108
USA

Index

Numbers in **bold** indicate figures.
Numbers in *italic* indicate plate numbers in the colour section